Unlearning Ableism

of related interest

The #ActuallyAutistic Guide to Advocacy
Step-by-Step Advice on How to Ally and Speak Up with
Autistic People and the Autism Community
Jennifer Brunton Ph.D. and Jenna Gensic M.A.
ISBN 978 1 78775 973 2
eISBN 978 1 80501 641 0
Audio ISBN 978 1 39980 411 0

Trans and Disabled
An Anthology of Identities and Experiences
Edited by Alex Iantaffi
ISBN 978 1 83997 080 1
eISBN 978 1 83997 081 8

Unlearning Ableism

The Ultimate, No-Nonsense Guide
to Understanding Disability
and Unlearning Ableism

Celia Chartres-Aris
& Jamie Shields

FOREWORD BY KEELY CAT-WELLS

Jessica Kingsley Publishers
London and Philadelphia

First published in Great Britain in 2026 by Jessica Kingsley Publishers
An imprint of John Murray Press

2

Copyright © Celia Chartres-Aris and Jamie Shields 2026
Foreword copyright © Keely Cat-Wells 2026

The right of Celia Chartres-Aris and Jamie Shields to be identified as the
Author of the Work has been asserted by them in accordance with the
Copyright, Designs and Patents Act 1988.

Front cover image source: adapted from iStockphoto® and Shutterstock®.

A CIP catalogue record for this title is available from the
British Library and the Library of Congress

ISBN 978 1 80501 875 9
eISBN 978 1 80501 876 6

Printed and bound in the United States by Integrated Books International

Jessica Kingsley Publishers' policy is to use papers that are natural, renewable
and recyclable products and made from wood grown in sustainable forests.
The logging and manufacturing processes are expected to conform to the
environmental regulations of the country of origin.

Jessica Kingsley Publishers
Carmelite House
50 Victoria Embankment
London EC4Y 0DZ

www.jkp.com

John Murray Press
Part of Hodder & Stoughton Ltd
An Hachette Company

The authorised representative in the EEA is Hachette Ireland,
8 Castlecourt Centre, Dublin 15, D15 XTP3, Ireland (email: info@hbgi.ie)

Contents

Acknowledgements

Celia: To the young girl who never thought she would be here alive to see these moments, yet alone achieve anything, there is a whole story to be written, never lose faith, you are the impossible girl.
An enormous thank you to my husband James, you seem to me to be, in every way, the visible personification of absolute perfection.
A heartfelt thank you also to my parents who, no matter what, always remained steadfast in their faith in me, showed me how to remain strong in the face of adversity, and always showed up with pride when I needed them.

Jamie: To the kid labelled 'special', the teenager struggling with his identity, and the adult who hated being Disabled, just because you couldn't see the stars then doesn't mean you won't reach for them now. Thank you to my lioness mummy and incredible daddy for being my first advocates, my first and last line of defence and for helping me to become the man I am today. And to my incredible partner, David Johnston, thanks is not nearly enough for the person who helped me find the strength to be unapologetically me. You are my rock, my bear, my support, and my world!

We both would like to thank everyone who has contributed to this book – your wisdom, experiences, and advocacy are truly paving the way for the generations to come. And a special thank you to David Shiels and our other close friends, who have been through the tears, tantrums, and many many edits, until the very end, helping us turn our vision into a reality.

PS, before we start...

We respect an individual's right to self-identify. Throughout this book, we use the terminology person with Disability, and Disabled person interchangeably to represent the diverse global audience we intend this book to reach. There may also be other points of language or terms you might not identify with that have been used, since we, and all of our contributing parties, have the utmost respect for the right of an individual to choose to identify and use the language of their preference in description of their own characteristics.

Foreword

BY KEELY CAT-WELLS

I still remember the first time I came across Celia and Jamie online. I was scrolling late at night, one of those 'just five more minutes' doomscrolls, and stumbled on a post they'd shared. It was sharp, funny, and unflinchingly honest. The kind of post that makes you stop mid-scroll and think, *Wow... I needed to hear that.*

Since then, I've been lucky enough to get to know them both. Individually, they're forces of nature, fierce, unapologetic advocates who aren't afraid to name what others tiptoe around. Together? They're a powerhouse pair with this rare ability to cut through noise, challenge norms, and invite people into a better way of thinking and being.

As a Disabled entrepreneur and Disability rights advocate, I thought I had a pretty solid grasp on ableism. I live it every day. But reading this book, I found myself underlining sentences, scribbling in the margins, and muttering 'oh, that's good' more times than I care to admit. This book is a mirror, a guide, and an important call to action.

What Celia and Jamie do so brilliantly here is take a subject that tends to terrify people because, let's be honest, nobody wants to 'say the wrong thing' and they make it approachable. Even funny. They don't scold; they invite. And then they challenge you to do better.

I've learned so much from them about leadership, about language, about unlearning the biases we don't even know we're carrying. Their advocacy has made me a better leader, a better ally, and, honestly, a better human. I know I'm not alone in that. This book will do the same for you.

This book is sharp, practical, and generous, with plenty of moments that will make you laugh, wince, and rethink everything from hiring practices to public policy.

I feel safer in a world where this book exists, because it means more people will finally start to see ableism for what it is: the biggest barrier of all.

So if you want to understand how systemic ableism harms all of us (and how to dismantle it), start here. Let this book challenge you. Let it change you. And don't be surprised when it makes you laugh out loud, too.

Because access isn't optional. Inclusion isn't a favour. And equity for Disabled people? It's long overdue.

CHAPTER 1

Unlearning Ableism:
The Diversity of Disability

> There is a misconception that Disabled people are some kind of rare mystical unicorns that only come out during full moons, that we are few and far between, hidden away in the shadows. This could not be more wrong. Disabled people are your friends, your neighbours, your colleagues, your customers. We are you.

Close your eyes, and picture a Disabled person. What do you see?

Like most people, you're probably envisioning a visible physical difference, something you can see, when the reality is that Disability is so much more.

Whether permanently or temporarily, we will all experience Disability at some point in our lives. To contradict societal misconceptions, 80% of people acquire their Disability at some point in their lifetime as opposed to the 20% of people born Disabled (Wheeler, 2022). You may break a bone, acquire a long-term illness, experience mental health conditions (yes, mental health is also included within Disability), all coupled with being in an ageing population. This is not intended to scare-monger, but if you think Disability doesn't apply to you, it may well in the future. Or it will affect a loved one. Disability is intertwined with human experience, so why do we not allow for the consideration of Disabled people?

Disabled people make up nearly a quarter of the population in the UK, 24% according to the Family Resources Survey (Department for Work and Pensions, 2023). That's over 16 million people, a number that is rising every year. Globally, the number of Disabled people is estimated to be 1.3 billion (World Health Organization, n.d.). Disability prevalence varies across different regions, reflecting demographic, social, and policy-related factors. In the US, more than one in four adults (28.7%) live with a Disability, as reported by the Centers for Disease Control and Prevention (2023). Within the European Union, an estimated 27% of individuals aged 16 and over, equivalent to about 101 million people, identified as being Disabled in 2023 (Eurostat, 2024). Similarly, in Canada, 27% of the population aged 15 and older, representing 8 million people, reported having at least one Disability (Statistics Canada, 2024).

However, due to equality disparities globally, access to healthcare or diagnosis, the definition of Disability, and data collection, the number of Disabled people globally is often disputed. Disability advocates and organisations estimate this number to be much higher than 1.3 billion, believing it to be larger than the population of China, which is 1.409 billion people (National Bureau of Statistics of China, 2024).

Statistically, we are the largest minority group.

Despite this, Disabled people are still having to navigate a society of which the very design excludes and disables. The societal knowledge gap around Disability has always been a vast chasm, where people are too scared to investigate the unknown. It is no wonder that society holds such misguided views on what it actually means to be Disabled, or how indeed the discrimination Disabled people face can be broken down. Society is inherently ableist. We are not educated about the history of Disability, our platform is consistently taken away from us and non-Disabled People incorrectly act or speak on our behalf, we are not consulted, we are not represented. We are living in a world which intends to promote surviving but not thriving.

But what does it mean to be Disabled? How do you define the lived experiences of over 1 billion people globally? Well, it's not an easy job, but we are going to try.

Have you heard of the Disability models? These are frameworks that seek to define and educate others about Disability. These frameworks create mechanisms that shape people's views, understanding, and perceptions of what it means to be Disabled.

Some models can positively lay the foundations to create inclusive law, policy, access, resources, support, and treatment of Disabled people; however, others further ostracise and perpetuate harm for Disabled people.

The two main models of Disability are the social and medical models.

The medical model of Disability

This model was christened in the early to mid-20th century, at a time when medical professionals were key decision-makers in diagnosing, defining, and 'treating' Disability. It was also a period when advancements in technology and medical science were bringing to light new treatments and ways to manage conditions. This model of Disability dictates that Disability is a component of humanity, to be treated and eradicated, a problem to be solved. It also reduces the human experience to the condition or impairment, failing to acknowledge societal barriers and systemic ableism. Under this model, if a Disabled person was not treated equally or included it was due to their Disability.

A small nod of appreciation must be given to the medical model. It paved the way for medical advancements and treatments and allowed researchers to gather valuable insights. However (we did say a small nod), without centring or encompassing those with lived experiences, a portion of these insights have now been proven to have detrimental repercussions – for example, the use of asylums, inhumane treatments, and forced terminations. This medical view of Disability didn't just define Disability among the medical community, oh no. It reinforced societal attitudes towards Disability that have arguably been there since the dawn of humanity. Disabled people are to be silenced, hidden away, cured, or ostracised. It influenced society to view Disability as a problem, something that we need to fix.

As you can imagine, this model of Disability is exactly the view of Disability we are trying to move away from. And what we should be moving towards is the social model of Disability (by the way, it's not just us; the United Nations also agrees!).

The social model of Disability

Surfacing during the late 20th century, this model stipulates that rather than viewing Disability as an entity to be cured, actually it is the intersection between our Disability and the societal barriers that disables a person (much better thinking, don't you agree?). The social model gained prominence thanks to the work of Disability rights activists and scholars. A huge contributor to leading this was Professor Mike Oliver, a Disabled academic. Mike coined the term 'social model of Disability' in 1983 (Oliver, 1983). Sadly, he passed away in 2019, but he left behind a legacy that challenges society to realise that *it* is disabling *us*. This model, and the work of Disability rights campaigners such as Judy Heumann, challenged the medical model view of Disability hoping to flip the narrative that had been written about us. Nothing about us without us.

The manual for removing barriers is centred around those with lived experience. Now we are writing our own narrative, as it should be. Ableism is a contributing factor that excludes and disables; where a non-Disabled person can navigate society freely, a Disabled person will encounter inaccessible buildings, inequitable healthcare and education – the list of barriers is endless. Disability is not the problem to fix; inaccessibility, ableism, and the underrepresentation rife within our society are the problems.

Of course, these two models are not the only models, but they are the most prominent within the Disability community. Other models are described below.

The charity model

This model views Disability as something to pity, and again rather than addressing inequities and inequalities, the solutions to address Disability centre around benevolent acts of kindness. It is as though Disabled people are all victims that society should feel charitable towards – Disabled people can't do it alone; they need non-Disabled knights in shining armour to save the day and rescue them from their tragic life. The charity model of Disability is one of the most criticised models of Disability. It focuses on what Disabled people lack, and mitigates their rights, opportunities, and their involvement in society. This model is often a wolf dressed in sheep's clothing, meaning it is inherently ableist. Understanding it helps us to understand how far we have come, where we are, and the mistakes of the past that we should not be repeating.

The biopsychosocial model

This model views Disability as an interaction between biological, psychological, and social factors. In other words, it takes parts of the medical model and social model while recognising mental health, emotions, genetics, internalised ableism, and other psychological factors associated with Disability. This model promotes a more holistic approach to Disability. While this model may seem on the surface the best of both worlds, it can also create the potential for blame. That blame is placed on an individual for not being 'mentally strong enough to manage their Disability' (even writing that felt ableist). It can also create additional ableist beliefs or stereotypes that Disability is just 'in a person's head'.

The rights-based model

This model focuses on Disabled people having equal rights across society, the same rights as non-Disabled people. Disabled people should be treated with respect and dignity, and be free from discrimination. This model focuses on protections and removing societal barriers so that Disabled people can be included in all areas of society. While this is a fantastic approach to ensuring the protection and inclusion of Disabled people, there are some who argue that it is unrealistic due to the inequality of access and the disparities in provision of care across the globe. This model also reduces Disability to one piece of an identity, overlooking individuals with intersecting identities who experience compounded discrimination.

But which model is right, and which is wrong?

Each model has its place, and without the progression through the models, we wouldn't have landed where we are today. Without the charity model, we wouldn't understand how far we have come and how far we have yet to go. Without the medical model, we wouldn't have the social model. Without either of these models, we wouldn't have the biopsychosocial model or rights model. People evolve. Attitudes evolve. Language evolves, and so do society's views of Disability. We don't know what the future brings and what new models lie in wait, ready to be shared with the world, but for now, it's important to know that each individual who has lived experience of Disability, or of being Disabled, will have their own view of what it means to them, how they want to self-identify, how they want to receive support, and how they feel about being a Disabled person. Therefore, it is up to the individual to decide, not a group, not a workplace, not another claiming to be 'an expert'. We told you that Disability is diverse, so if you are going to understand anything about Disability from this first chapter, understand its diversity, understand how to define Disability.

Defining Disability

In the UK, for example, the term Disability is defined under the Equality Act 2010. According to legislation, a person is considered Disabled if they have a 'physical or mental impairment that has a substantial and long-term (12 months or more) negative effect on their ability to carry out normal day-to-day activities'. It is important to note that the definition includes both visible and non-visible Disabilities, as well as conditions that may fluctuate in their impact over time. The purpose of this definition is to provide legal protection against discrimination, the provision of adjustments, and to ensure equal opportunities for individuals with Disabilities in areas such as employment, education, housing, and services.

The definition of Disability can vary depending on the country and context. In many countries, including the US, Disability is often defined by laws such as the Americans with Disabilities Act and the

Rehabilitation Act of 1973 (US Department of Justice, n.d.). According to these laws, a Disability is an impairment that substantially limits a person's ability to perform major life activities, such as walking, seeing, hearing, speaking, breathing, learning, and working. This definition includes people with 'physical Disabilities, sensory Disabilities (such as vision or hearing impairments), intellectual Disabilities, and mental health conditions'.

But the global consensus is that Disability refers to any physical, physiological, neurological, or mental condition which has a substantial impact on an individual's daily life.

It is also important to note that Disability is not solely determined by the presence of a health condition, but also by the interaction between the individual and society. This means that social and environmental barriers can contribute to the experience of Disability and impact the level of functioning and participation of Disabled individuals.

The notion of Disability has evolved over time to emphasise the importance of inclusion, accessibility, and equal rights for Disabled people; whether this is adhered to or not is another matter. When we define Disability, we are being asked to define diversity, but diversity is not one thing. Disability is not one thing.

Disability has no one appearance

There are many ways to experience Disability, from physical Disabilities to mental Disability, to chronic conditions, sensory Disabilities, neurodivergence, and so on. Disability encompasses a broad spectrum of lived experience. Disabled people can be white, Black, Brown, masc presenting, fem presenting, gender non-conforming, tall, short, slim, curvaceous...you get the picture. Disability has no one appearance.

There is no one experience

No two Disabled people experience Disability the same, and equally no two people with the same Disability experience it in the same way. Disability is uniquely personal to an individual. Their experience will be shaped by other pieces of their identity, environments, preferences, support, geography, and so on. While there are shared experiences between Disabled people and a deeper level of understanding and empathy towards another's experience, that person's experience of Disability is unique to them. Disability is shaped by many things.

Some Disabilities are visible

Some Disabilities are visible, meaning you will 'see' if a person is Disabled. This might be a person using a wheelchair, a walking aid, with a support animal, or the person may have a visible difference. A visible Disability does not mean a person will suddenly get the support or access they need. Disability being visible does not guarantee acceptance, support, or access. It also does not give you a right to stare or point.

Some Disabilities are non-visible

You will not always know just by looking at a person if they are Disabled. In the UK, Post Parliament (Kelly & Mutebi, 2023) reports that 70–80% of Disabilities are non-visible. In the US, the Centers for Disease Control and Prevention reports that 10% of Disabled people have outwardly visible Disabilities (as cited in Eisenmenger, 2020).

So, you will not always know if a person is Disabled and even if the Disability is visible it does not mean you will understand it. It is important to note that even a non-visible Disability can be made visible. For example, a visually impaired person using a screen reader or larger monitor can make their Disability visible to others. This might deter an individual from sharing or using the tools or the support they need. Just because you can't 'see it', doesn't mean it isn't real, or any less validated. You can't see gravity, but that doesn't mean it isn't there!

Disability can be permanent

Permanent Disability is long lasting or lifelong. Usually this means a person's Disability cannot be taken away with surgery, therapy, or medical intervention. The person's Disability will have a significant impact on their lives, and they may require specific support, adjustments, access needs, or alternative ways to engage. Permanent Disability does not mean a person is incapable or not deserving of opportunity or that they do not deserve the right to enjoy a fulfilling life.

Or it can be temporary

Temporary Disability is not lifelong and is only experienced by a person for a set period of time. This could be the result of a broken bone, sickness, pregnancy-related conditions, recovery from surgery, and so on. Temporary Disability can impact a person's movements, participation, and ability to perform tasks. It can change how they do things for a set amount of time, until they have healed and recovered. We are all one accident or sickness away from experiencing temporary Disability.

There is no right way to be Disabled and no wrong way to be

Whether a person is born with or acquires a Disability, it is important that we recognise there is no right or wrong way to be Disabled.

There is no magical handbook that suddenly tells us how to advocate, what adjustments/accommodations we need, or how to articulate our experience. Instead, we learn through trial and error.

We learn from having to navigate a disabling ableist society. Yet, we as Disabled people carry a weight or shame that it is our fault, that we should have said XYZ when we were being discriminated against, that we should try harder, as though the problem was even us in the first place. There is no right or wrong way to be Disabled – scream it from the rooftops, shout it from the hills. We need to stop placing unrealistic and unfair expectations on Disabled people. And we, as Disabled people, need to learn to stop carrying the burden of responsibility for a disabling ableist society.

Disability is one piece of our identity

A person's identity is made up of lots and lots of different things, but as a society we have a tendency to singularly label and categorise. We view Disabled people through a lens of everyone being the same, when the reality is that Disability is diverse, and it is shaped by all the other pieces of our identity. Our identity includes lots of things like race, class, sex, gender, age, sexuality, ethnicity, region, and nationality. Being Disabled is only one part of who we are; it is not our entirety. When you have met one Disabled person you have met one Disabled person – you will hear that a lot in this book. Disability is diverse, just as people are diverse.

Disability is intersectional

Disability does not discriminate. It is not restricted to one ethnicity, one race, gender, sex. Disability can be experienced by anyone at any given time, and it overlaps with every piece of a person's identity. This shapes a person's experience of Disability, creating instances of privilege and compounded oppressions. For example, a white Disabled woman will not experience Disability the same way as a Black Disabled woman. While the two women will have a collective experience of sexism, the white woman will not be judged by the colour of her skin, offering her some privilege which the Black woman is not granted. This does not make the white Disabled woman any less oppressed; it simply means that while she can empathise with the experience of racism, she will not herself experience it nor truly understand how it feels. Likewise, with a person with sight and a person without sight, the person with sight has the privilege of being able to see, whereas the person without sight does not. Admitting privilege is not an admission of guilt but rather an admission of understanding. I understand that my experience is different to yours.

Disability is human

As a society, we have the tendency to see Disability as this far away thing which does not directly affect or impact us, when in fact we are all just one accident or sickness away from experiencing Disability. As we age, we may acquire Disability or we may get sick, so rather than viewing Disability as a far-away thing we need to realise that Disability is an intrinsic piece of being human. It is encoded in our genes; it's in our DNA, passed down across the ages. Disability has always been here and will always be here because Disability is a part of the human experience.

We can't possibly have this discussion about Disability without talking about carers, an often-overlooked piece of the Disability conversation. Carers support, provide help, empower us, encourage us, and are there through the good, the bad, and the inaccessible – those unpaid and paid individuals without whom many of us wouldn't be where we are today.

But what is a carer?

A carer is someone who provides care and support to a family member, friend, neighbour, or relative who requires assistance to complete their daily tasks, that is not part of their paid work. A carer may provide support to someone for multiple reasons, not just Disability or neurodivergence. This includes temporary illness, an elderly person, someone with mental health challenges, reduced mobility, or an addiction, or they may just be keeping someone safe.

A carer may:

- provide support to somebody of any age, from children through to an elderly person

- also be Disabled themselves

- be of any age, from children through to an elderly person

- be full time, part time, or only when requested

- support with daily tasks such as getting out of bed, washing and personal care, financial affairs, food, taking someone to appointments, completing their errands, or socialising

- provide emotional support, companionship, socialisation, mental health support, or problem-solving skills.

66 I was a carer for my daughter, Lucy, when she became poorly at 14 years old until her death at 29 years. When you have a Disabled child from birth, often the parent(s) are made aware of services available for support for both the child and the parents.

However, when your child suddenly becomes unwell at 14 with an unrecognised disease/condition you are left floundering in the dark. I was working full time and was a single parent with an older daughter who needed me too. The whole system is so difficult to navigate. If I were asked for advice, I would say to seek out other families who have had success with negotiating with various different agencies. There is so much available provided you know how to access it. Lucy acted as an advocate for other Disabled young adults, for which she was awarded an MBE. She was passionate about ensuring that young adults and their families had adequate knowledge and knew how to put this into practice. Despite all her knowledge she often turned up at events (having made people aware that she used a wheelchair) and would be unable to get into the building or room. It was incredibly frustrating. It made us very aware that Disabled people are not always considered by society. 〞

– Kate Watts, carer

Carers are all too often under-valued and under-appreciated in the work and support they provide. Discrimination against carers is both discrimination against the Disabled community and the caring community, and therefore understanding how we unlearn the ableism within our biases, attitudes, and behaviours towards carers is essential.

Let's provide some perspective of the scale of this conversation:

- The International Alliance of Carer Organisations estimated that there were over 63 million carers worldwide (International Alliance of Carer Organizations, 2021).

- In Europe, 20% of the population identifies as a carer (European Foundation for the Improvement of Living and Working Conditions, 2021).

- Over 82 billion hours are spent each year on informal care for people with dementia in their homes (Wimo, Prince, & Gauthier, 2018).

- An estimated one in seven people is an unpaid carer while also being in employment (Carers UK, 2023).

With an ageing and growing population, rising social care costs, changes in social dynamics, and an increase in the Disabled population, these numbers are just going to get higher and higher.

Carers play a significant role in the lives of Disabled people and contribute to the broader understanding of Disability, ableism, and access through various lived experiences. They also have first-hand experience of the barriers that Disabled people face each and every single day and they too have their own challenges:

- Carers often face significant emotional and physical stress due to their caregiving responsibilities, which can lead to burnout and chronic health issues (Wisner, 2025).

- The economic burden on carers is considerable, with many facing reduced income and increased expenses (Wisner, 2025).

- Around 40.4 million Americans provide unpaid care for individuals aged 65 and older, with 32.9% of them reporting mental or behavioral health issues (American Psychological Association, 2020).

- Over half (55%) of family caregivers have been providing care for at least three years (Shuman, 2025), which increases the risk of physical and emotional burnout.

- A significant proportion of family caregivers, especially those caring for terminally ill or elderly relatives, experience post-traumatic stress disorder (PTSD), with 35% reporting depression and 70% experiencing anxiety (Braich, 2021).

- Twenty-five per cent of caregivers report significant difficulty accessing affordable and helpful support for their caregiving responsibilities (Family Caregiver Alliance, n.d.).

It's important to note that at times there can be tensions between Disabled people and carers. Now, we aren't talking about handbags at dawn here, but occasionally there can be differing opinions.

- Some Disabled advocates push for self-representation, believing carers should amplify Disabled voices, not speak for them. This perspective emphasises the importance of autonomy and ensuring that individuals with Disabilities have control over their own narratives. Carers, while often well intentioned, may inadvertently overshadow the voices of those they support, leading to tensions in advocacy efforts (Herr, 2016).

- Disabled advocates push for autonomy and self-independence, while carers, particularly family members, may restrict or discourage actions they themselves don't feel comfortable with. This dynamic can lead to conflicts, as carers' protective instincts might limit the personal growth and freedom of Disabled individuals. Balancing safety concerns with the individual's right to self-determination is a common challenge in these relationships (Maker, 2022).

- Disabled activists often feel that carers focus on a medical model lens, viewing Disability as something to be cured, rather than focusing on societal barriers. The medical model emphasises impairment and seeks to 'fix' the individual, whereas the social model highlights how societal structures and attitudes disable individuals. This fundamental difference in perspective can lead to misunderstandings and disagreements between Disabled individuals and their carers (Disability Nottinghamshire, n.d.).

- Some Disabled advocates believe that carers use outdated or ableist language, not listening to the individual or wider community. Language shapes perceptions, and the use of insensitive or inappropriate terms can perpetuate stigma. Advocates stress the importance of adopting language that reflects respect and aligns with the preferences of the Disabled community (Reynolds, 2018).

We are not here to referee these differences because, ultimately, the outcome should always be the autonomy of each Disabled person. While some Disabled people are able to express their wants and needs, others may not be able to or might struggle to do so, with their carer acting on their behalf. Perhaps this person does agree with the language being used, perhaps they understand how much this carer actually does for them and recognises that their intention isn't to offend but rather to support them in the best way they know how. After all, there's no course a person takes to become a carer; there are no qualifying conditions. People learn as they go, they adapt, they fight a broken system, and they do what they can. Now of course we recognise there are people employed to provide care, but for unpaid carers, a lot of the time they are thrust into the role.

There is space for those with lived experience and those who are carers to share their views and experiences; in their role as carers, they do experience ableism. They witness the inaccessibility, they hear the side comments, and they are the ones people seem to look at and talk to rather than addressing the Disabled person. They must be able to contribute to the conversation, and they must do so respectfully towards Disabled people. And equally, Disabled people must also respect carers.

Open dialogue is key.

Disability is beautifully and infinitely diverse

Everyone has their own unique lived experience. Lived experience will differ from person to person and even among those who may have the same or similar conditions. Each Disabled person should be viewed for who they are, an individual, not a stereotyped collective.

Close your eyes again, and picture a Disabled person. What do you see now? Are you beginning to recognise the diversity of Disability? Are you ready to now learn what shaped that view in the first place?

CHAPTER 2
Unlearning Ableism:
Defining Ableism

> 'I never would have guessed you were Disabled.' 'But you look so normal.' 'If you're blind where is your guide dog?' 'You are so clever, how on earth can you be dyslexic?' 'I've seen you walking, you don't need a wheelchair, stop pretending.' 'You have a job, so you can't possibly have ADHD.' 'Oh wow, you have a partner, and they're okay with it?' 'It must be so hard to be Disabled.' 'You're so inspiring.'

Ugh!! If we had a coin for every time a Disabled person heard comments like this being used so casually and without thought… we would be extraordinarily rich indeed. Time and time again these comments are thrown into conversation, idly and without consequence.

This is society's way of reminding us that 'to be Disabled' is to be viewed and treated differently, and that it is justified for people to behave accordingly. This is an example of ableism. These hurtful phrases, although seemingly innocent to the user, can actually reinforce the charity model of Disability. 'Oh, you achieved something and that is amazing because you are Disabled.' This comment, which you might think is a compliment, actually reduces an individual to their Disability and makes them inspiring not because they achieved, but because they are Disabled. Welcome to unlearning ableism!

So, what is ableism?

Ableism refers to the discrimination or prejudice against individuals with a Disability, or the belief that Disabled people are inferior to those without Disabilities. Because of this belief, Disabled people are marginalised, prevented from opportunities and participation, or denied basic rights and accommodations. Sounds straightforward, right?

Unfortunately, it is not that simple. It is hard to summarise ableism in a single sentence. How do you summarise in words that which has, and continues to have, a significant detrimental impact on the lives of Disabled people globally?

The Oxford Review (n.d.) defines ableism as, 'discrimination in favour of the able-bodied'.

The irony, of course, is that this definition is quite ableist. It creates the idea that every Disabled person does not have use of their body. It implies that to be Disabled is to not be able.

However, a more accurate definition of ableism would be the systemic oppression of Disabled people. Ableism restricts Disabled people's movements, autonomy, rights, and inclusion across society. Ableism shapes people's view of Disability, in turn leading them to act with bias, stereotype, and to exclude and discriminate.

As a society, we are innately ableist, automatically designing spaces, products, and services in a way that excludes Disabled people. Our workplaces, healthcare, and education systems are not inclusive or representative of Disability, and yet we continue to talk about making change. But the same belittling undertone is that to be Disabled is to be treated differently.

Ableism is ingrained in language that speaks to us as if we are less than or at times more than, simply due to a piece of our identity. Treatment that seeks to wrap us up in cotton wool or remove us completely. Biases and stereotypes that fail to grasp the complexity or the diversity of Disability. A society that is unaware of what it means to navigate systemic ableism. Unless you're a Disabled person/person with Disability, or you're in proximity to Disability, you probably aren't even aware of ableism, or even what it means to be ableist. This emphasises yet again that we haven't always, and in many cases still don't, teach young people about ableism, workplaces don't always include it in their training or policies, doctors don't mention it or discuss its impact, and even Disabled people do not always understand or get the opportunity to learn about it.

If society is perpetuating the notion that Disabled people are not part of 'normality', and continues to exclude and segregate us and have us believe we are less than the ideal of normal, is it any wonder we are in the position that we are in?

But how exactly does ableism manifest?

Aggressions (micro and macro)

Data from the World Health Organization (2022) reported that over 15% of people with Disabilities globally face macroaggressions in the form of physical barriers, and a study conducted by the Disability Rights Education and Defense Fund (Jammaers & Fleischmann, 2024) found that over 50% of Disabled individuals reported experiencing microaggressions regularly.

Ableist microaggressions manifest as patronising or condescending actions, behaviours, and language. People's well-meaning intentions can often be deep rooted in ableism. Telling someone, 'I don't see you as Disabled', 'I never would have guessed you had a Disability', and other comments which downplay or erase a piece of a person's identity is ableist. It is the belief that Disability has one appearance, one universal experience. This utterly mitigates the fact that Disability is diverse; there is not one set 'appearance'. Disability is both visible and non-visible, sometimes both. It can be both permanent and temporary, sometimes both. There is no one experience; even if people have the same Disability, their experiences will be unique to them.

Microaggressions, either verbal or non-verbal, cause harm, offense, or discomfort to another person. In the context of Disability, this could be microaggressions such as asking invasive questions about a person's Disability – 'How do you have sex?', 'How do you go to the bathroom?' Such questions only serve personal curiosity and are in no way supportive or inviting to the individual. Microaggressions can also include how you act or behave around Disabled people, for example suddenly changing your tone as though you are speaking to a child on realising they are in fact Disabled, or ignoring the Disabled person speaking to you and instead speaking to their companion.

Macroaggressions, on the other hand, are a lot more obvious. They are much larger in scale and include things such as the designing of inaccessible buildings or environments, segregation of Disabled people in education, discrimination against Disabled people, or disparities and inequities within healthcare. We could go on here, but as you read this book you will learn just how ableist macroaggressions institutionalise ableism, making it part of our society. It is also important to note that aggressions, whether micro or macro, are aggressions. Even if you view or consider something to be a microaggression, it can and might feel like a macroaggression to the individual experiencing it.

When you opt to downplay or erase Disability, you are telling us that we do not conform to your idea of Disability, an idea that is incorrect anyway. When you treat us differently because we are Disabled, you are displaying microaggressions.

Assumptions

In a 2020 survey, 38% of Disabled people reported that they were often assumed to be less capable of handling social or professional responsibilities than their non-Disabled peers (Office for National Statistics, 2021). People make ableist assumptions about Disabled people, their needs, abilities, worth, and capabilities. We assume because we do not know, and we're not taught about Disability. Assumptions prevent us from recognising the diversity of Disability and the contributions and value of Disabled people. If we assume every Disabled person is the same, we overlook intersectionality and how intersecting identities shape a person's experience of ableism. Don't assume, ask. Ask how you can support a Disabled person; don't think you know what they need or what they are going to be capable of. Assuming anything about a Disabled person without first speaking to them, knowing them, and asking them, is ableist. You cannot assume the needs of a Disabled person simply by looking at them.

Attitudes

The National Center for Learning Disabilities and Understood, in an annual survey, found that 'just 30% said they "feel strongly" that they're able to successfully educate students with learning Disabilities' and 'just half of the surveyed teachers said they "feel strongly" that students with learning Disabilities can perform at grade level'. 'As such, researchers found that a significant share of educators held several common misconceptions about people with Disabilities. A third of respondents blamed students' learning or attention issues on laziness, a quarter believe such issues can be outgrown, and another quarter pin ADD and ADHD on bad parenting' (Keierleber, 2019).

Ableist attitudes are a reduction of a Disabled person's identity, isolating out their Disability as their only factor, the only thing worth knowing about them. These attitudes create an environment for marginalisation. To be marginalised is to be overlooked, excluded, and treated as less. It is not having equal and equitable access to resources, opportunities, rights, and protections. Ableist attitudes towards Disabled people can present as pity, treating them as inspirational due to a piece of their identity, not for their actions or accomplishments, and it can take the form of stereotyping or making presumptions of someone's 'capabilities'. Ableist attitudes stem from a lack of education on Disability, and ableism that we cyclically emanate into society.

Bias

A 2020 study by Harvard University's Project Implicit found that 60% of participants showed implicit bias against Disabled people (Ratliff & Tucker Smith, 2024).

Ableism is rooted in bias. 'Oh, Disabled people can't do this.' 'We don't have any Disabled team members.' 'They can't be autistic because they are verbal.' This bias changes the way we interact with and view Disabled people. Bias occurs because of negative attitudes and beliefs that a person holds. This bias can often result in treating Disabled people with pity or sympathy: 'Oh, poor Disabled person, life must be so hard for you.' It is believing that Disabled people are inferior or that we are less capable than our non-Disabled peers: 'Well, how would they be able to do it? They're Disabled.' Bias can also show up when people perceive Disability to be entirely physical.

The vast majority of people have a distinct assumption that Disability is only something that can be instantly seen (visible Disabilities) and don't acknowledge non-visible Disabilities. People can also opt to use language which implies that Disability adjustments are 'special treatment'.

Bias can be implicit or explicit. Implicit bias is subtle or unintentional, such as assuming a d/Deaf person cannot hear anything at all, a blind person cannot see at all, or a wheelchair user cannot use their legs at all. We subconsciously have a biased view of what Disability should be, and create bias about how a person should look, behave, or even communicate. Explicit bias, on the other hand, is intentional. It is choosing not to hire a person because you know that they are Disabled. It is purposefully setting out to exclude and harm Disabled people. Explicit bias is easier to recognise, while implicit bias is typically harder to unlearn because we don't know that we are doing it.

Remember, bias is not always conscious. We are conditioned to perceive Disability to be one thing: a wheelchair user. This is as a result of the universally used symbol of Disability, found on parking, websites, bathroom doors, and even bumper stickers. But Disability is diverse. Not all Disabled individuals require mobility aids such as wheelchairs. World Health Organization (n.d.b) data suggests that around 80 million people globally, or 1% of the total population, rely on wheelchairs for mobility. When considering wheelchair users as a subset of the Disabled community, they represent roughly 6–7% of all Disabled individuals globally, which means that this symbol is not representing 93–94% of the Disabled community.

Beliefs

According to Scope's 2014 survey, 67% of people reported feeling uncomfortable talking to Disabled people (Scope, 2014).

Ableist beliefs form our opinions and view of Disability. As a society, we have set an unrealistic standard of what we consider to be normal. People create a comparison between Disability and normal – 'They're not Disabled, they're normal' – implying that to be Disabled is some undesirable, ugly trait. Or because a Disabled person interacts or navigates things in a different way, we automatically believe them to be not as capable, not as worthy, not as socially acceptable. We set Disabled people up to fail by believing they are going to fail, they aren't going to be as good, as capable, or as hard working.

Discrimination

Research by Scope shows that 54% of employers surveyed said they had concerns over a Disabled employee's ability to do the job, and this affects their decision to offer a Disabled person the job (Scope, n.d.b).

Discrimination, in all areas of identity, is defined as the unfair, unjust, and prejudiced treatment or exclusion of an individual, or groups based on characteristics such as race, gender, sexuality, religion, Disability, and other characteristics. In a legal context, discrimination is the unfair and unequal treatment of individuals or groups based on 'protected characteristics'. Disability discrimination is running rife through our societal cultures around the world and is being allowed to do so. In a survey conducted by the Disability Unit UK (2021), 52% of Disabled respondents reported having experienced mistreatment due to their Disability. Discrimination is found in workplaces, due to actions, behaviours, or when companies do not provide adjustments/accommodations or fail to provide equal and equitable opportunity for development or promotion. Discrimination happens in education, healthcare, transportation, travel, and through social and attitudinal barriers. In other words, it is blooming everywhere, in every aspect of our lives.

Inaccessibility

In a 2023 survey by the Business Disability Forum, half of Disabled employees reported that their workplace was inaccessible in terms of physical spaces and accommodations (Business Disability Forum, 2023).

Society has been designed for the non-Disabled and neurotypical – it's as simple as that. Everything, from our infrastructure right through to the design of websites, is not accessible for a lot of Disabled people. According to a 2025 report by WebAIM, 94.8% of the top one million webpages had accessibility issues (WebAIM, 2025).

From the outset, entrenched in our societal structures, Disabled people are excluded. We are not provided with the same opportunities to participate, engage, or connect. When people think of accessibility, they typically think of physically accessing a building, accessible bathrooms, lifts, or ramps. They don't remember to also think about digital accessibility or the accessibility of events, travel, healthcare, and so on. Workplaces and communities play a pivotal role in contributing to ableism. The failure to provide accessibility, or the failure to consider accessibility, is ableism.

We need only to look at the design of society to realise that Disabled people are treated less favourably. They are not considered when it comes to designing a new office, launching a new product, or even when you yourself post a message on social media. We have all heard the horror stories: a wheelchair user not having access to the building, guide dogs refused entry to public spaces or Disabled people struggling to gain and retain employment, no consideration to the fact that not everyone has the privilege of sight, sound, mobility. Ableism is rampant, thriving, and ready to raise its head at any given time.

Not everyone interacts with the world in the same way, yet we continue to exclude, and fail to provide opportunities for Disabled people to belong. We currently lie in a state of reactivity not proactivity, but we have to be forward thinking. We cannot continue on this cycle of waiting for discrimination to happen; we have to step in, and step up to make changes.

Lack of adjustments and accommodations

A report by the European Union Agency for Fundamental Rights (2020) highlighted that one in four workers with Disabilities in the European Union reported experiencing difficulties in obtaining the accommodations needed to perform their job.

Not providing adjustments and accommodations is the failure to provide an equitable experience for Disabled people. While international Disability law determines what is reasonable, there are many instances where companies fail to offer or promote adjustments and accommodations. Many people are also not aware that adjustments and accommodations go beyond the workplace. If you are holding an event, creating a webpage, or creating marketing content, not providing accessible options or the means to request them excludes Disabled people. Society has drifted towards this notion of set-templating, cookie-cutter normality, and we all think and act the same way. No. Not everyone learns, thinks, communicates, or navigates the world in the same way, and failing to consider this creates barriers which exclude and discriminate.

Language

Numerous studies, and declarations of lived experience by Disabled people, demonstrate the inherant ableist language on social media platforms such as X (formerly Twitter) and Instagram (Jerez, 2024).

We acknowledge that language is an ever-changing, ever-evolving concept; however, the language we continue to use when talking about Disability or the experience of Disabled people has remained so far behind the inclusive progression of our dictation. How many times have you used Disability slurs, said 'Wow, that's mental', 'I was so blind to it', 'They're just slow'? In education, we label Disabled children's needs as 'special' or across society people perceive the words Disabled and Disability to be negative. Rather than utter these words, they opt for fluffy sugar-coated language: 'differently abled' or 'different abilities' or 'diverse abilities'. This is language used to make others feel comfortable, not the Disabled person.

Ableist language evokes strong reactions and for good reason. It reduces us and our experiences to an entirely negative space, with the undertone of disrespect, burdening, negative projections, and hurtful intent whether conscious or not. This is not, as we hear all the time, 'wokeism gone too far' or an 'infringement on freedom of speech'. Unlearning our language that we have grown up with and is ingrained within us is no simple feat; it takes time, we make mistakes, and we have to undo everything we know to create new habits. But this isn't an excuse for failing to do it all. We must educate and be educated by others with lived experience.

Inspiration porn

The term 'inspiration porn' was coined by Australian Disability activist and comedian Stella Young. Stella used the term to describe the objectification of Disabled people as tools to inspire non-Disabled people (Young, 2014). 'You are so inspiring', 'You are so brave', and 'You are so inspiring for pushing through this.' This is inspiration porn. Our Disability is placed above our identity, our achievements, and our skills. You could be a lawyer, and when you tell some people that you have a Disability, they will be proud of you for simply saying you have a Disability, not because of your achievements. That's not inspiring; that's empowerment for the individual disclosing. It's inspiring for other Disabled individuals to see such empowerment. But for the person without a Disability, what have you learned? The person is Disabled. Do we need a marching band to mark this inspirational moment? You set your expectations so low that when we do something absurd like tie our shoelaces or hold down a job, you pat yourself on the back for recognising how hard it must be for that poor Disabled person. The only person who is benefitting from this exchange is you. You may think you have the best intentions, but without really knowing someone, their achievements, their values, and their beliefs, can you truly call them inspirational?

Picture this. If we told you a father saved his son and died in the process, you would think, 'What an inspiration.' But given context, that man was Darth Vader. He murdered, butchered, and wiped out the Jedi Order. But without that context, you didn't know that. If you want to feel better about yourself, rather than getting off comparing yourself to Disabled people, start unlearning ableism – it's much better for you.

Stereotypes

Scope, a UK-based Disability equality charity, found that over 72% of Disabled people had experienced negative stereotypes related to their Disabilities in the previous five years (Scope, 2022). We generalise about Disability, creating false perceptions and ideals of what it means to be Disabled. 'Well, you can't be a wheelchair user because I saw you walking yesterday.' We stereotype because we aren't aware, we don't understand the complexity of Disability, we only know what we have seen or been taught, and we know that's not readily available or adequate. Phrases like, 'Oh, they all are suffering' and 'All Disabled people need help' generalise and overlook the experience of individuals.

Stereotyping is patronising and negative and creates a false narrative of what it means to be a Disabled person. When you allow your bias, either consciously or unconsciously, to inform your view of Disability, you have just stereotyped. Stereotyping is incredibly harmful; it perpetuates negative beliefs and assumptions and reinforces false perceptions of Disability. It is believing that blind means total vision loss, that d/Deaf means you cannot hear anything, or that to be Disabled means you are less 'capable'. These stereotypes create a society that holds the view that to be Disabled is to be one thing. Meeting one Disabled person is meeting one Disabled person. Just like our unique fingerprints or neurological profiles, no two Disabled people are the same. Making false judgements or allowing your own bias to inform your view of Disability and the way you treat Disabled people is harmful.

Are you aware of ableism?

Ableism is systemic and unlearning it requires an individual to be increasingly aware of their own actions and behaviours. Ableism has created a power imbalance for Disabled people. It has restricted our ability to influence, make change, and advocate for ourselves. This imbalance of power is a driving factor of sustaining the marginalisation of Disabled people.

It is worth noting that even Disabled people themselves are not always educated on ableism, or, because of the diversity of Disability, have only experienced a small portion of the endless possibilities ableism has to offer. Disabled people are also not taught ways to manage ableism, how to challenge behaviours, and how to overcome discrimination, so this only further fosters our own internalised ableism, which can cause long-lasting psychological trauma.

Internalised ableism is the cost Disabled people pay when navigating a society not designed for them – a cost unwillingly and unknowingly paid. Internalised ableism is the direct impact ableism has on a Disabled person. It shapes our view of Disability, affects our self-worth, advocacy, and our mental health. We will further explore internalised ableism later in this book.

Ableism is a major factor when it comes to a Disabled person feeling a sense of belonging, feeling accepted, and even feeling supported. How can we embrace our authentic Disabled self when society seeks to treat us as less or, in some cases, as inspirational? Society is working against us, and we internalise these thoughts to work against ourselves. Can you imagine how exhausting that is? We navigate this society and when we speak out against ableism we are often viewed as over sensitive or angry. We are labelled as snowflakes, woke, or challenging. But if you strip it down, all we are asking for is to be included, to not be treated as an exemption or afterthought.

Now you may be thinking to yourself, well of course I agree that Disabled people shouldn't be punished, ostracised, or treated unfairly, but these decisions are not made by me individually; they are made by governments, leaders, policies. And yes, you would be right, they are, but as individuals we also play a fundamental role in unlearning ableism. You might have:

- used outdated offensive language

- made a biased judgement about a Disabled person/person with Disability

- told someone they don't look Disabled or treated them differently, without ever being invited to do so

- created an inaccessible product or service

- shared content online that was not accessible

- operated with exclusionary social practices

- displayed biased attitudes

- stereotyped somebody

- denied someone adjustments and accommodations.

Ableism constructs barriers that hinder our full participation in various aspects of life and act as a driving factor to our social exclusion. The list of ways in which as individuals we contribute to ableism is endless, and even the best intentions might have ableist undertones. The good news is you're not alone. We have all done it at some time or another, we have all witnessed other people doing it, and we all have gaps in our understanding about how to address or even stop it. To unlearn it, we must first understand its influence and grasp on society.

The Ableism Cycle

Ableism is systemic. It is ingrained in the structure and design of our society, woven into its very fabric, and it thrives within our communities. To understand its influence and impact on society we use the Ableism Cycle, a resource and tool we created to educate others about ableism.

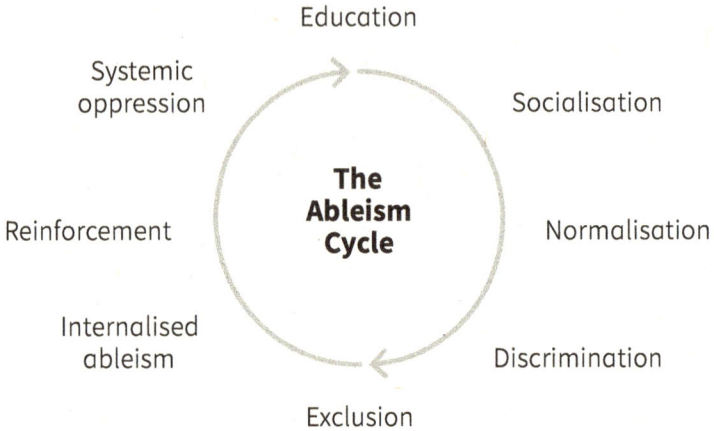

Education

Systemic oppression

Socialisation

The Ableism Cycle

Reinforcement

Normalisation

Internalised ableism

Discrimination

Exclusion

Education

- Young Disabled people navigate an inaccessible ableist education system, designed for the neuro-majority and the non-Disabled.

- It is an education system that historically has segregated and treated Disabled people as 'special'.

- Non-Disabled young people witness this segregation and exclusion, learning that this treatment of Disabled people is acceptable and normal. They witness the segregation of Disabled people from an early age in turn grow into adults who design and create an environment, products, and services that are inaccessible and exclude Disabled people.

- There is inadequate training on Disability within education, limiting the support a child receives. There is often a lack of accessible resources and support, resulting in parents and caregivers having to fight for their child's right to education.

- This exclusion continues across education, from preschool to university, with barriers presenting themselves to Disabled people and preventing them from achieving or obtaining an adequate education.

Socialisation

- A lack of education and understanding of Disability causes people to learn from sources closer to home, such as friends, family, and media.

- As a society, we are influenced by what we view and deem as 'normal'. We learn what is perceived to be normal, desirable, or attractive qualities and traits. This often leads people to believe that difference is not normal and does not bring value.

- We learn from others how to treat and act around Disabled people. Adults are seen to treat Disabled people with pity or through a charity lens – 'That poor wee child' – and young people inherit and adapt these behaviours, informing their beliefs and the way they themselves treat or view Disabled people.

- A lack of representation and false representations of Disability in media, in leadership, and across society also leaves people to formalise their own thoughts and views. Disabled people are made out to be victims, or Disability as an undesirable quality. Disabled people are portrayed in movies with lives that are tragic and unfulfilling and there is a complete failure to include Disabled people in lead charter roles or as the hero. It's easier to label the person with facial scarring or with missing limbs as the villain, portraying Disability as undesirable.

- People hear words and phrases used in everyday conversation and they cling to them and repeat them in their own vocabulary – words which are offensive, outdated, and ableist in nature. Words like 'crazy', 'lame', and 'retarded' carry hurt and pain for many, but are used so casually in conversation, in music, on TV, and as part of our everyday conversations.

- A lack of understanding and representation of Disability has led people to believe stereotypes or make assumptions about Disabled people, in turn leading them to act unintentionally ableist when they do meet a Disabled person.

Normalisation

- Society sets the standard to design for the non-Disabled, that to be a non-Disabled person is more capable, more hardworking, adds more value. The narrative is that to be Disabled is problematic, causing us to exclude because why would we design for Disabled people? They are not our ideal customers (insert eye roll here).

- Cultural standards normalise the idea that Disability weakens a person, that to be independent and capable is the standard everyone should achieve.

- The ableism in our language is considered generational, where the harm of certain words and phrases is downplayed and those questioning the language are labelled as woke, outspoken, or sensitive.

- Socialised ableist values and beliefs become ingrained in our systems, policies, laws, healthcare, education, and workplaces, continuing to further exclude Disabled people across society. People design and create in the way they have been taught, continuing an inaccessible cycle which ends with Disabled people excluded and discriminated against.

Discrimination

- When society is designed to not include you it's inevitable that you as a Disabled person will experience discrimination. As mentioned earlier this can be direct discrimination or indirect. The cycle of ableism is designed to oppress and discriminate Disabled people, keeping us from achieving, from belonging, and from being accepted.

- This discrimination leads to lack of opportunities, 'We don't hire Disabled people', biased hiring decisions, 'Disabled people are not as hard working as non-Disabled people', and other ableist mishaps that both directly and indirectly discriminate against Disabled people.

- Discrimination is not always experienced in a professional setting either, as many Disabled people have been denied friendships, relationships, and autonomy of their bodies simply because they are Disabled. There is a belief that to be Disabled means you are not capable of understanding relationships, your body, your choices.

- Historically, discrimination has ensured that Disabled people are not given the same equitable opportunities as non-Disabled peers, ensuring our exclusion across society.

Exclusion

- Exclusion can take many forms: physical, digital, social, economic, institutional, and so on. Exclusion denies Disabled people access, opportunity, and participation across society, whether that is being able to bank, shop, connect, or even work.

- This exclusion can drive Disabled people to mask or hide their Disability when applying for jobs, dating, and so on. We do this because we believe it safer to hide our Disability than risk a repeat of the past, rather than experience further exclusion – already planting the seeds of internalised ableism.

- Exclusion can impact a person's mental health, leaving them feeling isolated, lonely, or desperate. In turn, this can cause a person to numb or hide the pain with drugs or alcohol and can lead to mental health challenges.

- Exclusion pushes Disabled people to the outskirts of society, further marginalising and ostracising them. It ensures that Disabled people can never truly participate and instead normalises ableism and sets the scene for internalised ableism.

Internalised ableism

- As mentioned earlier, internalised ableism is the cost Disabled people pay when navigating a disabling ableist society. In terms of the cycle of ableism, internalised ableism plays a fundamental role in continuing to oppress Disabled people.

- Internalised ableism leads Disabled people to accept and, in some ways, support the ableism ingrained in our society.

- What better oppresses a group or community than to have them question their own worth and value? That is what internalised ableism does. It costs a Disabled person their acceptance and shapes their experiences and, just like the example given earlier, we accept because we do not know any different, and because society reinforces the belief that to be Disabled is not attractive but is a problem to be solved.

Reinforcement

- Across society, ableism is reinforced and strengthened by other forms of oppression. Oppressions such as racism, sexism, homophobia, and classism support and uplift each other, ensuring that individuals remain powerless and marginalised.

- Despite the incredible work of Disability advocates across the world, we still are moving at a snail's pace towards creating a society that is inclusive and accessible for Disabled people. Accessibility is claimed as a cost; Disabled people are seen as a burden and unlikely to be a service user or customer. The idea that Disabled people can't make decisions, apply themselves, or engage or succeed is reinforced.

- Reinforcement solidifies the socialisation of ableism. It validates the normalisation of ableism, and it cements the discrimination and exclusion of Disabled people by justifying inequitable treatment. It reinforces that being Disabled is a problem in society.

- Ableism is ingrained in every piece of our society. We have been saying this, but we hope by now you can understand just how deep this problem is. Reinforcement ensures that ableism remains a systemic oppression, supported and propped up by other systems of oppression.

Systemic oppression

- Ableism is behind every workplace door, every poor portrayed misrepresentation of Disability in media, behind that well intended act of charity, and the use of derogatory language meant to offend and upset a Disabled person. Every piece of our society is rooted in ableism. Think of it like a big weed that has rooted itself across the fabric of our society.

- Systemic oppression means that ableism remains large scale, affecting every single aspect of a Disabled person's life, whether it's at school, college, work, or visiting the dentist. Ableism is there, lying in wait.

- Our culture's ableism is an inherently harmful concept that perpetuates systemic oppression. This belief is devaluing the inherent worth and dignity of Disabled people and denying us our basic human rights, equitable opportunities, and the right to equal participation. Accessibility and inclusion are a right not a privilege, a legally binding principle that appears to have been forgotten.

- When society chooses to not include, design, or consider Disabled people, it contributes to this cycle by ensuring Disabled people remain oppressed and excluded. There is no recognition that one day these very people might be the ones on the other side of the oppression, the ones needing the accommodations.

The Ableism Cycle is cyclical, with each step feeding into the next, each series of events happening repeatedly, like being trapped on a giant hamster wheel, only this hamster wheel is not alone, oh no. It is sitting in the path of other forms of oppression, other systems that are marginalising groups and communities.

Now you might be wondering, how can ableism cause so many problems for Disabled people and still go unaddressed? You have just asked yourself the same question millions of Disabled people have asked themselves. Why does this cycle continue? How is it allowed to continue?

As a singer once sang, 'You can run, you can hide, but you can't escape…ableism.' Okay, ableism was not the follow-on word, but the point is this: ableism is everywhere, and you cannot continue to bury your head in the sand. To not stand up to ableism is to contribute to the exclusion and discrimination of Disabled people. Unlearning ableism means looking at yourself and recognising your contributions; it means understanding that Disability and ableism can impact a Disabled person. A fabulous way to do this is to start using Spoon Theory.

Spoon Theory

Trying to discuss how Disability and ableism can impact a person can be difficult. How do you explain your everyday to a person who does not yet understand Disability? Thankfully, Christine Miserandino (2003) has described her individual experiences of exhaustion while navigating society with a chronic autoimmune disease. She uses a concept known as Spoon Theory, which has now been widely adopted as a way to talk about the experience of Disability.

So, what is Spoon Theory?

1. Imagine everyone starts each new day with 20 spoons. Each spoon represents the energy you have for the day.

2. The tasks we complete throughout the day cost an individual a certain number of spoons. For example, brushing your teeth costs a spoon, going to work costs a spoon, eating breakfast costs a spoon – see where we are going with this? Everything costs a spoon. Every task we complete requires

spoons, so there is no escaping spoon usage. Some tasks require more spoons than others. For example, you might spend more spoons travelling to work on a day where your train or bus is late than on days when it is on time, which is rare, we know.

3. Non-Disabled people might make it through the day with just the right number of spoons to complete everything they needed to do. But for Disabled people, activities and tasks that would cost a non-Disabled person one spoon could cost twice as much. Think of a journey to work for a non-Disabled person using a train. They can arrive at the station, get their ticket, and board the train. But a wheelchair user must check ahead of time if the train station is accessible, if there is someone to help get them on and off the train. This journey is costing the Disabled person more spoons than the non-Disabled person.

4. This additional spoon usage is not only afforded to travel, but also across other aspects of the day. A visit to a shopping centre might cost a non-Disabled person two spoons, but for an autistic person it might cost four spoons due to the additional sensory and communication barriers. Everyday tasks and actions that would cost a non-Disabled person a few spoons can often mean double the cost for a Disabled person. And while certain tasks will cost more spoons for a Disabled individual, it does not mean every single Disabled person will use the same amount of spoons for said task. Remember, Disability is diverse; so are our needs.

5. Disabled people tend to run out of spoons before the day is out, either from personal challenges or because of ableism. This could mean we run out of spoons and have to go into the next day with a deficit of spoons. Running out of spoons is a fast way to experience burnout.

Ableism costs Disabled people spoons that non-Disabled people would never have considered or imagined. It's important to recognise that a Disabled person's day to day can look very different from a non-Disabled person's, since the vast majority of products and services are designed for the non-Disabled, without accessibility in mind. This in turn creates barriers that exclude Disabled people. Across the day, Disabled people have to navigate these barriers, costing yet more spoons.

When we also consider the intersecting identities of Disabled people, these spoons may disappear even faster. Navigating a society not designed for you is exhausting, mentally and physically, so wasting spoons on the ableism of others is not what we want to be doing! But sadly, the reality is that this is the cause of burnout and internalised ableism. Unlearning ableism can help remove some of this additional spoon usage.

Ableism intersects with every piece of a person's identity

Ableism intersects with other forms of discrimination, such as racism, sexism, homophobia, and classism, resulting in even more profound marginalisation for individuals with intersecting identities. Disabled people from marginalised communities often face compounded discrimination, further exacerbating the challenges they already confront. We wake up to ableism. We navigate ableism throughout the day and go to bed exhausted from it. Now add racism, sexism, homophobia, transphobia to that person's day, when they are already navigating a society that historically has overlooked and created power imbalances. We will explore this much more in our intersectionality chapter and in other areas of this book.

" Whenever we talk about ableism, it's important to talk about it in the context of other intersecting forms of discrimination. When we think about how we challenge ableist systems or behaviour, we also need to think about the other factors that lead to the oppression of an individual. We need to address the presence of 'intersectional ableism'. We all have multiple identities, whether that's around race, gender, belief, and so on. Two of my identities are that I am both a person of colour and a Disabled person. I've seen how ableism compounded with racism can exacerbate exclusion, creating further barriers to healthcare, education, employment, and social participation.

It's my view that all systems of oppression are deeply intertwined, shaping policies and practices that disproportionately harm Disabled people. Here are three examples of what I mean by 'intersectional ableism'.

We know that Disabled people of colour face higher unemployment rates due to workplace discrimination and systemic barriers to education and career advancement. Recent research from the National Disability Institute in America (2019b) shows the intersection of race and Disability as being one of the key drivers of poverty.

Throughout history, Disabled women have faced forced sterilisation and the denial of reproductive autonomy – policies rooted in both misogyny and eugenics. Even today, only nine EU countries criminalise forced sterilisation as a distinct offence, while 13 allow it to be performed on individuals with Disabilities – and in three of those countries that includes minors (Amoakuh, 2024).

Access to inclusive healthcare is another critical issue. LGBTQIA+ [lesbian, gay, bisexual, transgender, queer, questioning, intersex, asexual, and others] individuals already face discrimination in medical settings, and this is amplified for those who are Disabled. Research produced by the European Disability Forum (Uldry, M. & EDF Women's Committee, 2022) shows that medical professionals may invalidate a Disabled person's queer identity or make inappropriate assumptions about their ability to engage in relationships. So when we think about ableism, we need to think about how it often sits at the intersection of other forms of injustice – and if we cannot just challenge one form of injustice, we need to challenge them all. 〝

– James Lee, Disability advocate

You have taken your first steps to unlearning ableism

We get it, not everyone likes being called out. But if we don't start challenging and unlearning ableism, we won't ever break its cycle. Addressing ableism requires a collective effort to challenge negative attitudes, dismantle systemic barriers, and foster inclusive and accessible environments. It involves educating ourselves and others about Disability rights, advocating for policy changes, promoting inclusive practices, and actively listening to and centring the voices and experiences of Disabled people. By taking accountability of our own learning, and working towards creating an accessible inclusive society, we can dismantle ableist barriers and create an environment that embraces and values the diverse abilities and contributions of all individuals.

This book is your guide to unlearning ableism, helping you understand the complexity of ableism, how it manifests, and just how it contributes to the exclusion of Disabled people.

You can't run from ableism, nor can you excuse yourself from it. It's time to pull your head out of the sand.

CHAPTER 3

Unlearning Ableism:
Internalised Ableism

> 'It's me. I'm the problem; it's me! Or rather, it's my Disability. It makes me weak. It's embarrassing, it's shameful. I hate it. I hate me. I hate being Disabled.'

Spending your life navigating a society not designed for you is hard. When all you want to do simply is exist, but yet all around you is barrier after barrier, another form of ableism, and another reminder that to be Disabled is to be a problem.

Many Disabled people don't view the inaccessibility or ableism as the problem; we view ourselves as it. Our conditions, impairments, neurodivergence, and differences make us the problem. Society doesn't exactly tell us otherwise; in fact, it just reinforces this belief.

Lack of representation tells us that Disabled people are not of value, that Disability is not attractive, and that we won't achieve because we are Disabled. Inaccessibility tells us we are an afterthought, that to be Disabled means we are a problem to be solved, that Disability is the reason for our discrimination and exclusion.

Yes, society doesn't do much other than remind Disabled people that we are the problem, and internalised ableism thrives on it. With 50.3% of Disabled people experiencing internalised ableism at least once a week, the reality for Disabled people is that no matter where we hide we cannot escape ableism or internalised ableism (Disabled by Society, 2024).

What is internalised ableism?

Ableism, as we are learning, is rooted within society, and we all contribute to it. Internalised ableism, on the other hand, is rooted within an individual. Internalised ableism happens when Disabled people begin to adapt and absorb the ableism they are experiencing externally across society. As we absorb this ableism we internalise it, and it begins to influence and shape our view and experience of Disability. 'This is what it means to be Disabled,' we tell ourselves.

Internalised ableism is the cost of ableism and, as we are learning, ableism isn't a rare experience for a Disabled person. Disabled by Society (2024) reports that 46.6% of Disabled people experience ableism at least once a week, while Scope (n.d.) reports that 87% of Disabled people say that these ableist experiences adversely affected their daily lives.

Studies also show that individuals who internalise stigmatising beliefs about their Disability are more likely to experience poorer mental health, which can be linked to negative psychological outcomes like depression, anxiety, and lower self-esteem (Corrigan & Watson, 2002).

Imagine that every day when a person wakes up, they have to wear a pair of glasses – that's everyone, everywhere. The glasses you wear have a slight smudge in the bottom corner and no matter how much you have tried cleaning them, that smudge doesn't budge. The smudge stays there. You get used to the smudge thinking everyone must be the same, right? Yes, you might choose not to go to certain places because of the smudge, or you might not speak to others about the smudge, and because no one else is talking about theirs, why would you? Your smudge-stained glasses are just what it means to be you. The smudge, which at first was annoying, you have grown used to. It has become part of your daily routine. You learn to live with the smudge; the smudge is 'normal', isn't it?

One day, you and a friend decide to swap glasses. While trying theirs on you notice they don't have a smudge in the corner of theirs. Your friend doesn't have to react to things in certain ways, they don't have to watch out for things, they are smudge free. This is a bit like internalised ableism. As Disabled people we spend our lives navigating a society where we are excluded and treated as 'less than'. We begin to accept this as our reality. We begin to accept that the ableism we experience is our normality, and just like that smudge on those glasses, we are seeing things through a distorted lens. We have accepted the ableism because we do not know any other way. This allows our internalised ableism to manifest and shape our view of Disability. We believe and accept the bias, mistreatment, and exclusion we experience, simply because we are so used to it, just as we got used to the smudge on our glasses.

Without education about ableism and internalised ableism, we believe the distorted view that 'being Disabled' makes us the problem.

But just as seeing the world through your friend's lens helped you see clearer, learning about ableism and internalised ableism can help change a Disabled person's view of Disability, and themselves.

> 66 Internalised ableism made me feel broken for existing normally. I hid my Disability (a congenital birth defect) for 17 years

until the age of 27. It took me two decades to understand that Disability is not outside the norm; it is the norm. The problem is that society has shrunk the definition of normal, which leads to bias, judgement, and, worst of all, self-doubt for anyone existing outside that false norm. The most sinister part of internalised ableism is that it has nothing to do with your actual capacity or lived experience and everything to do with society's misunderstanding and ignorant classification of something it truly knows nothing about. When that internal ableism comes about, remember to ask yourself, 'Do I actually feel this way or did society teach me to feel this way?'

– Chris Ruden, amputee, Type 1 diabetic record-holding powerlifter, motivational keynote speaker

Experiencing ableism over a sustained period of time begins to affect our self-esteem, our self-worth, and our self-value. These experiences stack on top of each other like a game of Jenga, shaping our view of Disability and what it means to be Disabled. Most of the time we aren't even aware it's happening. Unknown to us, the trauma of these experiences remains with us even after the moment of ableism has passed. And just like Jenga, internalised ableism lies ready to offload at any given moment, impacting and shaping us in diverse ways:

Heightened emotions: Internalised ableism can lead to heightened emotional responses from Disabled people. Not having an outlet or a way of processing the emotional trauma of ableism can create increased feelings of anger, frustration, or sadness, and lead to outbursts or emotional responses that are uncharacteristic of the person.

Self-worth and self-value: Internalised ableism can make a

Disabled person feel as if they are weak, that their Disability is embarrassing; that they are less than, less capable than others. This impacts the way we view ourselves and our Disability. It tells us that Disability makes us inferior, that being Disabled means we cannot achieve.

Self-advocacy: Internalised ableism can feel like an inner monologue running through our head, a voice telling us not to share our Disability. It tells us to deny or reject offered support, and to not ask for the adjustments and accommodations we need. This in turn can prevent Disabled people from receiving the support they need.

Mental health: When internalised ableism has a negative impact on a Disabled person's mental health, this can lead to things like low self-esteem, anxiety, depression, isolation, self-doubt. When seeking support from medical professionals about internalised ableism, it can be difficult due to a lack of understanding and resources.

Isolation: Internalised ableism can lead a Disabled person to isolate themselves from friends, family, and support networks. The feeling of not belonging and the fear of ableist experiences repeating themselves can lead a Disabled person to withdraw from activities, and refuse to leave the house or socialise.

Addiction: Internalised ableism can cause a Disabled person to look for coping mechanisms or ways to mask their feelings of shame or anger. This can lead Disabled people to self-medicate with alcohol or illegal substances, creating a cycle of shame and addiction and placing them in vulnerable situations.

Self-harm/suicide: Internalised ableism can contribute to self-harm or suicidal thoughts for Disabled people. The psychological toll of internalised ableism can leave a Disabled person feeling despair, lost, shame, hopelessness, and as if they are incapable of love, success, or happiness.

There's no off switch, no reset, no getting over it, just like ableism.

Many Disabled people experience ableism, completely oblivious that it has a name. According to Disabled by Society (2024):

- only 14.1% of Disabled people were taught about ableism in education

- only 15.2% were taught about ableism in the workplace

- 62.4% of Disabled people have had to teach themselves about it.

With limited resources and learning opportunities it can make it hard for Disabled people to realise the impact or effects of internalised ableism. A study by the Council on Quality and Leadership (Friedman, 2024) found that while 72% of Disabled professionals believed they understood ableism, only 48% could accurately define it.

Health professionals don't discuss or consider the impact of internalised ableism, nor do they understand the impact of Disability beyond a medical model view. A study published by the American Academy of Pediatrics (Ames *et al.*, 2023) found that caregivers of children with medical complexity and Disability reported experiences of Disability-based discrimination in healthcare. Themes identified included lack of clinician knowledge, clinician apathy, and clinician assumptions as drivers of discrimination, leading to limited accessibility to care and substandard care.

Yet society does not teach Disabled people about internalised ableism, and none of us discuss it being a contributing factor to the mental health of Disabled people. Research by Yale School of Public Health (2022) reported that ableism is a significant barrier to mental health care for Disabled people.

We have to remember that society isn't as open to discussing mental health as we may claim it to be.

The mental health stigma

Historically, speaking about mental health carried a stigma. People thought it was a sign of weakness, and carried with it a sense of shame. These are learned behaviours, which told men that speaking about their mental health made them less masculine, and told women that if they shared, it made them emotional. A study by the American Psychiatric Association (2024) showed that three in five people living with a mental illness did not seek support due to concerns about how they would be perceived by others. That stigma is still present – the stigma around mental health still impacts. As time progresses, we are witnessing changes and a shift in attitudes and perceptions. People are now destigmatising and normalising conversations around mental health. But we are not all the way there.

Unfortunately, the stigma of speaking about mental health is still ingrained in us, with many still finding it embarrassing, uncomfortable, or difficult to open up. We can then add Disability to the equation, and the unique challenges that come hand in hand with this.

Evidence suggests that 30% of people in the UK with long-term conditions also experience mental health problems such as depression and anxiety (Cimpean & Drake, 2011), while in the US, a study by the Centers for Disease Control and Prevention (2024) found that 32.9% of Disabled adults experienced frequent mental distress. This is why when we discuss the health and well-being of Disabled people, we cannot do so without addressing internalised ableism.

Mental health and Disability are part of the human experience, overlapping and co-occurring. We need to make internalised ableism a part of the mental health conversation. We need to be creating spaces that don't just talk about mental health, but provide adequate, accessible resources about internalised ableism and mental health. These should be spaces where health professionals feel comfortable to address the internalised ableism in the room, and where individuals with lived experience can feel safe to share their experiences.

Sadly, this is not the current experience. In many instances when Disabled people have advocated and spoken up about ableism or inaccessibility, or have asked for support, we have often been met with silence, discrimination, or fresh ableism. This sends us back into a loop of internalised ableism. It is as if we are expected to simply be okay with being excluded.

People are shocked that we dare to speak up, we dare to say 'no more'. People expect us to just be okay with being Disabled by society. It is because of these experiences when we have been silenced, called woke, labelled dramatic, needy, rude, troubling, or painted as an angry Disabled person, that often we do not say anything. Our internalised ableism tells us it's better to say nothing than risk a repeat of the past. Self-doubt is guided by fear, and steered by past and current trauma that shaped our internalised ableism.

Internalised ableism is internalised oppression. This is why we must remind ourselves that the Disabled experience is heavily impacted and influenced by ableism. Internalised ableism is the cost.

Internalised ableism isn't the same for every Disabled person. It's personal, and how a person experiences internalised ableism will be unique to them. It's also important to note that every Disabled person experiencing internalised ableism will be struggling with their mental health. Some individuals will have found ways of managing or have support systems in place. Each individual, just like Disability, has their own experiences of internalised ableism.

Lateral ableism/projected ableism

Disabled people are not exempt from ableism, and, in many cases, it is the projection of ableism from others in the community that can have the deepest impact on our internalised ableism. Have you heard the expression 'hurt people hurt people'? The same can be said of internalised ableism. An individual who is experiencing ableism can begin to project this onto others.

Consider a Disabled person who has struggled with their own internalised ableism. This has manifested in a way that they now consider the word 'Disabled' a negative word. When they witness other people self-identifying with the word 'Disabled' their response is to tell the person that Disabled is a negative word, and instead they should refer to themselves as a person with Disability.

While this is an ongoing debate within the many communities that exist of Disabled/people with Disabilities, we need to acknowledge that by telling others how to self-identify we are subjecting that individual to potential trauma. We do not know the reasons why a person chooses the language they do to self-identify; it is their right and we do not need to know. But what we do know is that self-identifying and the language we choose to use often come with their own challenges, confusion, and struggles. Finding the language that feels right for us is like trying assorted styles. Sometimes the style we choose today doesn't feel right tomorrow, and equally choosing the right style takes time, trial, and error, and usually some regrettable choices along the way.

When we project onto others and challenge their self-identity, we are invalidating their experiences, their journey, their lived experiences. Doing this can have a lasting impact, causing these people's internalised ableism to dissociate. This in turn can impact their sharing again. As the individual who made them question themselves, you too will have been through a journey of finding the right language for you at one time or another. Remember the confusion? Trying on different labels and trying to find the right one? The frustration? The lack of clarity? The voice of internalised ableism along the way reminds you not to say something because of what happened before, or what you heard others say. It's a difficult journey, so why would we want to subject someone to trauma?

So how does a Disabled person overcome internalised ableism?

We wish we could say here is the answer, but sadly there is no one answer because internalised ableism doesn't simply go away. It stays with us. It is the cost of ableism. All we can do is learn to manage, advocate, and find ways to support ourselves. Here we provide some of the tips we ourselves have used to support our own journey of unlearning internalised ableism.

Journalling
Keep a journal, and we don't just mean old-fashioned pen and paper. We mean, find the most accessible way for you to journal. This could be videos, voice notes, written notes, or even drawings. Whatever medium you choose, journal about your day, your week, your feelings, your worries, your challenges, or even about the ableism you have

experienced. This can be a form of therapy for many Disabled people, helping to express and articulate thoughts and feelings we may not have fully processed. It's also a fantastic way to dump out some of that internalisation. The thing you wanted to say at that moment, write it down. Type it. Draw it. Sign it. Scream it. Whatever way you approach it, do it for you.

Self-care

On the harder days, internalised ableism can make it feel physically impossible to get out of bed, to eat, to shower or even dress. It can make us want to hide away from the world, neglecting our needs and not advocating for ourselves. In these moments, our internalised ableism acts as an inner saboteur. Exercising, getting out of the house, speaking to someone, eating a balanced diet, nurturing your mental health, and setting boundaries are so important when prioritising your self-care. Plan, set yourself daily goals, and place reminders around you to encourage you to take care of yourself. Neglecting our needs only feeds into our internalised ableism and if we do this over a sustained period our mental health will struggle further, leaving us vulnerable, isolated, or depressed. So, make time for you. Set boundaries for yourself, and others. Set goals, no matter how big or small. Celebrate the wins. Find the time to prioritise you because you are the priority here.

Charities and non-governmental organisations (NGOs)

Being around people who get it can create a safe space to open up and share your experiences or feelings. Many charities and NGOs have set groups, forums, resources, and support. These spaces can provide a safe haven for those wanting to connect with other Disabled people, seek advice, or simply feel part of a group that 'gets it'. People who have been there. The good news is that there are many in-person and virtual communities set up, so you can find the most accessible ones for you. The sad news is there are so many amazing organisations that are doing incredible work across the world that if we began listing them, we would run out of pages. So instead, we encourage you to take a moment and google Disability charities and NGOs in your area. Review the results and utilise the incredible workers and volunteers who are helping create psychologically safe spaces for people to connect, learn, or meet others in their community.

Networking

The internet has opened up the world to us, with a special thanks to social media. Social media has enabled people to create communities, groups, clubs, and networks that connect like-minded individuals – people with shared hobbies, interests, or passions. Whether it's a blind/visually impaired community group, an attention deficit hyperactivity disorder (ADHD) network or a support group, a potential community could be a few searches away. Choosing which social media platform to use will be dependent on your preferred social media usage and what is most accessible for you.

Whether it's Facebook, Instagram, X, or LinkedIn, always remember to keep yourself safe online. Do not share personal data such as your address, credit/debit card information, phone numbers, and so on. And please only share what you feel comfortable sharing. You are the expert of your own lived experiences. But there are many other Disabled people out there who are the experts of their own lived experiences, individuals who will have shared experiences of ableism and internalised ableism, people who will get it. Connect, engage, and always stay safe.

Not sure where to start? Join Disabled Professionals on LinkedIn, a group set up by us to help Disabled people from across the world to vent, share, learn, support, and provide meaningful connection.

Reframing

One of the hardest things we can teach ourselves is to reframe. This involves countering negative thoughts or feelings with positive reinforcement. It can be tough trying to reframe the thoughts of shame or embarrassment, or the feeling that your Disability makes you a problem. But, over time, this reframing can help put things into perspective and provide some much-needed validation. For example, someone might think, 'My Disability makes me the problem.' Counteract this thought with, 'Society is not designed for me; this does not make me the problem.'

'I hate being Disabled' could be reframed as: 'Being Disabled does present challenges, but it does not define me as a person, or my value.' Focus on the positives, what you can control, not that which you cannot. And we get it, it can be cheesy at first, but, over time. reframing can be a great tool in your arsenal. It also can help us take a step back from an ableist or inaccessible experience and realise that we aren't the problem; it is the lack of education, accessibility, or understanding of society that is the problem.

Words of affirmation

You are your own worst critic. We all are our worst critics. We judge ourselves more harshly than others ever will. Internalised ableism will have us believing the worst about ourselves. It is easy to listen to this monologue and fall victim to believing; believing you are less, that you are weak, that you are the problem. In these moments, it is harder to push these thoughts and feelings aside than affirm them.

This is why it's paramount that we learn to love ourselves, which is one of the hardest things we can ever learn to do. Learning to accept yourself, being kind, and reminding yourself of just how incredible you are is something that we should all strive to achieve. Every day you get out of bed, you navigate a disabling society, you experience ableism from every direction, and you continue to do this each day. Yes, we waste a lot of spoons, but we also keep showing up. We may stumble, we may waver, but we show up time and time again.

You are a problem solver – you have to be in a society not designed for you. Yes, it's not fun, it's horrible, it affects us, but we are stronger than anyone else around us realises, than even we know. We continue doing all this, while our internalised ableism throws spanner after spanner, hoping for us to hand in the towel and accept its ableist narrative. Sometimes we do, we give in and believe the internalised ableism, but we get back in the saddle. You are powerful. It might not always feel like it, but you are. You overcome the oppression of society, the oppressions of internalised ablism, and you need to acknowledge this.

Find the time to give yourself credit. Remind yourself of your strengths. Be kind to yourself. Leave a message that is accessible to you, something that you will come across daily. Let that message be an affirmation. You deserve to be affirmed. Internalised ableism wants us to loathe and hate ourselves, so learning to love yourself won't be easy. But it all starts with learning to be kinder.

Don't compare

Society throws around the word normal as though it is a definable, reachable target. People perceive Disability as substandard, unnatural, not normal. We hear it when they describe non-Disabled people as normal. This false perception or idea of normal is learned behaviour that makes us compare ourselves to others. People who are not yet Disabled, aka non-Disabled people, have set the standard. It is a standard that is biased and discriminates us from the offset. Recruitment processes which aren't accessible, events that aren't accessible, inequitable workplaces, and so on, designed by non-Disabled people and not representative of Disabled people. But if we fail to address the inequities, we experiencing it will result in us comparing ourselves to others, meaning we don't fit the normal way of doing things, but the so-called normal way of doing things sets us up to fail, and we are not comparable.

So, please stop comparing yourself to others, whether Disabled or not yet Disabled. Your experience or Disability is unique to you, and comparing yourself to others only sets about an unfair outcome for everyone. People are unique. And so in comparing ourselves to others, however hard it is not to, we need to remember that equity means recognising we do not all start from the same place in life. We each have our own unique circumstances and experiences, and we are all diverse, intersectional beings. We cannot be compared because we each are fabric cut from different cloths.

Therapy or counselling
A safe, supportive environment can be incredibly beneficial to help explore and understand your internalised ableism.

This could mean exploring coping strategies, creating self-awareness and self-compassion, or helping to identify, understand, and get to the origins of your internalised ableism. Seeking help is a personal decision. If you are having negative thoughts, or are in distress, or finding it difficult to manage day-to-day because of internalised ableism, we implore you to seek support as soon as possible. If you need to speak to someone sooner, please consider using 24/7 support helplines.

Celebrate the wins
Positive reinforcement works by improving our self-esteem and by boosting our confidence. By celebrating both the minor and major wins you are actively positively reinforcing yourself, which given the nature of internalised ableism can be a beacon of light. Each win

is evidence of your resilience, your hard work, and your strengths. It also allows you to take a moment to reflect on something you might have missed or purposefully avoided. Celebrate in the way that makes you happy. Affirm yourself. Whether it's a snack, a gift, a day out, whatever makes you happy. Celebrate the wins.

To Disabled friends

We know that managing internalised ableism is an ongoing process. There are no quick wins, no magic wand, and no one-size-fits-all solutions. Experiment with different techniques, therapies, or self-care to find what works best for you and what feels most comfortable. You are never alone in this, even when at times it might feel like it.

> 66 For too long, I sought validation in the eyes of others, chasing approval, measuring my worth by the words and expectations of people who never truly knew me. I let their opinions shape my confidence, their judgements dictate my happiness. But no matter how much I changed, how much I achieved, it was never enough. Because the truth is, external validation is a moving target; you hit one mark, and another appears.
>
> The turning point came when I realised this: I will never find true fulfilment if I keep looking for it outside myself. Self-acceptance isn't about proving anything to the world; it's about embracing who I am, as I am. The scars, the struggles, the victories, the failures, all of it belongs to me. And that is enough.
>
> We live in a world that thrives on comparison, on likes and applause, on the illusion that we must be something more, something better, to be worthy. But the only validation that truly matters is the one we give ourselves.

I no longer seek permission to feel confident, to be proud, to take up space. I define my own worth. I validate myself. And in doing so, I have found a freedom that no amount of external approval could ever give me.

So, if you're waiting for someone to tell you that you're enough, stop. Look in the mirror. Say it to yourself. And believe it. Because you always have been. You always will be. 99

– Amit Ghose*

To organisations

Support your employees to learn about ableism and internalised ableism. Develop your health and well-being plans to include internalised ableism. Consider offering support for Disabled colleagues to speak to therapists, coaches, or counsellors. Talk about mental health but in doing so discuss internalised ableism. Start making mental health a priority for your organisation, not just another buzzword to fluff up your culture.

To educators

Please teach your students about ableism. Talk about internalised ableism. Talk about feelings and the importance of expressing these feelings. Provide learning material in your libraries and classrooms. Read books that represent Disability. Encourage self-advocacy and please ask the young person how they want to self-identify, and for the love of inclusion, please use the term they choose.

* Read more about Amit's story at https://talestoinspire.com/amit-ghose

Internalised ableism isn't going to go away. We do not have enough resources or understanding available to support the millions of Disabled people impacted by it. That's why we need to normalise education and conversations about ableism. By understanding and educating about ableism, Disabled people can begin to understand how this is impacting them. They can begin to understand the internalisation they are harbouring; they can begin unpacking their internalised ableism.

By creating accessible resources and making internalised ableism part of the mental health conversation we can begin to finally provide support and guidance for Disabled people who have spent too long believing that they are the problem, when we now know they aren't the problem; ableism is.

CHAPTER 4

Unlearning Ableism:
Intersectionality

> 'I'm not just Disabled...' 'I'm not just a woman/man/trans...'
> 'I'm not just Straight/Gay/Lesbian/Bi...' 'I'm not just White/
> Black/Brown...' 'I'm not just one single thing...' 'My identity
> is so much more...'

Disability can be experienced by a person at any given time, regardless of whether they are male, female, trans, asexual, non-binary, straight, gay, lesbian, or bi. It does not matter what a person's skin colour is or whether they are rich or poor. Disability is a universal experience, and it does not exist as a monolith. Disability encompasses a wide range of identities and experiences. There is no one way to be Disabled. There is no one appearance. There is no one experience. Disability can and will continue to be experienced by individuals from all walks of life.

But Disability is just one aspect of a person's identity; it is not their entirety. A person's identity is made up of lots of different things: gender, sex, sexuality, race, ethnicity, culture, neurodiversity, Disabilities, socio-economic status, religious or spiritual beliefs, and so on.

Each of these pieces intersect and intertwine, leading to instances of additional privileges and power, or causing further disadvantage, discrimination, and compounded oppression.

When we talk about the Disabled experience, we cannot do so without recognising that each person's experience of Disability is unique to them. To truly understand and value the diversity of Disability, intersectionality and intersecting identities have to be part of that conversation. When they are not, we aren't having the right conversation, and we are going to be excluding large groups of people.

But what is 'intersectionality'?

The term 'intersectionality' was introduced to the world and coined by Black scholar and legal theorist, Kimberlé Crenshaw. She wrote:

> The problem with identity politics is not that it fails to uncover oppression, but rather that it often fails to see the ways in which various forms of oppression intersect. The intersectional experience is greater than the sum of racism and sexism; it is a unique form of discrimination. (Crenshaw, 1989)

Society has historically viewed systems of oppression, such as racism, sexism, homophobia, biphobia, and transphobia, as separate entities, independent in their discrimination. Crenshaw argued that by doing this we fail to understand that these systems of oppression do not exist in isolation but rather they are co-occurring and interconnected. This means that these oppressions aren't experienced as two separate things, but rather they combine to create unique outcomes:

- additional privileges

- compound oppression.

In the 1990s and early 2000s, intersectionality was adapted by various groups, advocates, and activists from LGBTQIA+, Disability, feminist, and Indigenous communities.

But what is a system of oppression?

Systems of oppression are created when a dominant group has social, economic, and political power over another. They make decisions which directly impact and affect the lives of those without power, which creates a power imbalance. White heterosexual males have traditionally held power. For evidence of this you only need to look at the boards of most global organisations, where white cisgendered males hold the majority of positions of power. There is no representation, but instead an untrue, unrealistic mirror of the society in which they operate.

Society itself has been built on the blocks of white supremacy, capitalism, patriarchy, and other interconnected systems that have further discriminated, excluded, and ostracised individuals, groups, and communities. For example, ableism is systemic oppression. It is created because Disabled people do not hold power, and the very design of society and treatment from others in society keep them from holding significant power. Disabled people are then excluded as the dominant group in society; non-Disabled people are not excluded, and things are designed for them. This in turn creates a power imbalance and systemic oppression of Disabled people. Systemic means it affects the entirety of our society.

Other systems of oppression can include:

- **Sexism:** Discrimination based on sex or gender.

- **Racism:** Discrimination based on race or ethnicity.

- **Ageism:** Discrimination based on age.

- **Classism:** Discrimination based on social class or economic status.

- **Homophobia:** Discrimination against individuals based on their sexual orientation.

- **Transphobia:** Discrimination against transgender and gender non-conforming individuals.

- **Religious discrimination:** Discrimination based on an individual's religion or beliefs.

This list is not exhaustive.

A Disabled person won't just experience ableism but rather they will experience this co-occurring with other systems of oppression and, as we said, this in turn can create additional privileges or compounded oppression. But what do we mean by compounded oppression and what do we mean by privileges?

Compounded oppression

Compounded oppression refers to the ways a person can experience multiple forms of discrimination simultaneously, creating unique experiences and outcomes. Outcomes may include additional bias, additional barriers, and not being able to use systems that are meant to support but have not been designed to accommodate intersecting identities.

Think of an online support group for women. The group is open to women, but for a Disabled woman, if the platform is not accessible then they are going to be excluded. While the group was designed to support women, it further marginalises Disabled women.

A Black Disabled woman might experience both sexism and racism, which will create unique challenges for them. But this experience will not be the same as that of a white Disabled woman or a Black man or a white trans woman.

Compounded oppressions are created when systems of oppression support and reinforce the other.

Privileges

Spoiler, we all have privileges, but when some people hear this, they find it uncomfortable. They associate privilege with money, owning fancy things, or being born with a golden spoon in their mouth, but although this does include some instances of privileges, it is not the full picture. Privileges are unearned advantages or benefits that individuals or groups enjoy simply because they belong or were born into a dominant group. Admitting privilege is not this big bad thing that many people make it out to be, but the reality for many Disabled people and non-Disabled people is that they feel uncomfortable when they hear it. Feeling uncomfortable with something is a result of us not understanding it or fearing its outcome. But what kind of privileges can a person have?

- **White privilege:** The benefits and advantages a person receives simply because they were born white. This includes things like not being racially profiled, or a lack of white representation in media.

- **Male privilege:** The benefits and advantages men have over women and non-binary individuals. This includes pay disparities and less scrutiny for showing assertiveness.

- **Class privilege:** The benefits and advantages afforded to a person for belonging to a higher socio-economic class. This includes being able to afford private education, housing etc.

- **Heterosexual privilege:** The benefits and advantages afforded to people living in a heteronormative society. This includes things like not having to come out or not having marriage equality.

- **Non-Disabled privilege:** The benefits and advantages afforded to people who are not born with or acquired a Disability. This includes things like not having to worry about accessibility or internalised ableism.

- **Cisgender privilege:** The benefits and advantages afforded to those who are born to those whose gender identity matches the sex assigned at their birth. This includes things like not being misgendered.

We all have privileges

- If you have sight, you have privilege which someone without sight does not have.

- If you can hear, you have privilege which someone without hearing does not have.

- If you can speak, you have privilege which someone who is non-verbal does not have.

- If you have a house, you have privilege which someone without a house does not have.

See where we are going with this? Privilege is not a bad thing; it is merely being aware of the advantages you have been afforded which others have not been. It is not about blame or pointing fingers; it's about recognising our advantages and understanding others' disadvantages to help create empathy and understanding.

66 Intersectionality is critical to understand and appreciate because 15–20% of the global population is neurodivergent. This figure includes many people from a large array of backgrounds, religions, races, ethnicities, cultures, genders, and identities. The support we need as neurodivergent individuals varies not just from person to person but also culture to culture. Additionally, there are many barriers we encounter not faced by Caucasians, such as racism and xenophobia and fears of being treated more harshly in encounters with law enforcement. There is also much less access for Disabled persons of colour to assessments/diagnoses, mental health care, educational and employment opportunities, and housing.

From my experience, it is also much harder to connect with other people, as a Disabled person of colour, even within the neurodivergent community itself, meaning that I often encounter loneliness, depression, isolation, and alienation. I see intersectionality like a dating app. The more filters you have (diverse race, gender, ethnicity, etc.), the harder it is to find matches or people who connect with you. As a Chinese-born, neurodivergent, Jewish adoptee, I face this problem a lot. I have friends within the neurodivergent community who can't fully empathise or appreciate the barriers and trauma that exist when growing up in a xenophobic society as an Asian, or the isolation that comes with being told to 'go back to your own country'. It has been hard existing as a neurodivergent Jew during the Hamas/Israel conflict because I have seen many of my neurodivergent friends abandon me, and, rather than being supportive, act with hostility and anti-semitism.

Ending on a positive note, being a Chinese-born, neurodivergent Jew has given me a very different perspective on life, society, and identity. I can empathise with a greater number of people. I can use my experiences to inspire other Disabled people of colour to come forward and tell their story, thus breaking the chain of stigma and ableism that often afflicts multiply marginalised communities. 99

– Ben VanHook, a Chinese-born, Jewish, AuDHDer (autistic and ADHD)

Intersecting identities

We cannot hope to understand the diversity of Disability without understanding the framework of intersectionality and the diverse intersecting identities of people. Intersecting identities focus on the individual components of identity rather than the systemic impact of their actions.

A person might identify as a Black Disabled man, gay, and an immigrant. These identities create a unique experience for the individual which shapes the person's experience. Another person might identify as a white person with Disability, straight, and a national of the country they reside in. These identities create a unique experience for this individual.

- Intersecting identities are the specific identities an individual holds.

- Intersectionality is the framework used to help us understand how these identities interact to create compounded oppressions or privilege.

It is important to acknowledge and understand the significance of intersectionality and its origins. Too often the word is thrown around by people idly and without thought of its wider meaning.

We must understand the historical significance of the systems of oppression and their impact on the rights of Disabled people if we are ever to unlearn ableism. Disabled people with intersecting identities have often been left at the mercy of these oppressive systems, and in order to move forward we must learn from our past, or we will be doomed to repeat it.

Shared lessons from the past

Throughout history, movements like the Civil Rights Movement, the Feminist Movement, the Disability Rights Movement, and the LGBTQIA+ Rights Movement sought to fight for equal rights, justice, and protections for groups. Each of these movements was sharing a common goal, to dismantle barriers that create inequitable and unequal treatment and the need to create a world where individuals are valued for who they are.

Systems of oppression are cut from the same cloth.

Imagine a single piece of tie-dyed fabric. Think of how the tie-dye creates vibrant swirls of colour, those swirls of colour creating distinct sections. You would almost think this single piece of fabric had been created with lots of different pieces of fabric, but it has not; this is one piece of fabric, created using the same tie-dye process. Now imagine each section of that tie-dyed piece of fabric represents a different system of oppression, such as racism, sexism, or ableism. Although these systems have things that make them distinct, if you pull at the thread of one you will find it impossible to unravel without unravelling them all.

Throughout time, social rights movements have sought to overturn these systems and have shared lessons. Each movement helped to build on the lessons of those that came before, the sacrifices, the victories. Now, we are not going to give you a full history lesson here, as that's what we have our history chapter for, but it is important to understand how movements have supported each other across history and how if we are ever to dismantle them, we need an intersectional approach.

The Civil Rights Movement (1950s–1960s) worked to dismantle racial segregation and end the discrimination of African Americans. It laid the foundations for Disability rights activists by highlighting the need for equal treatment for all marginalised groups. The Feminism Movement, particularly from the 1960s onwards, significantly influenced Disability rights activists by highlighting the need for autonomy, bodily integrity, and reproductive rights (Evans, 2003).

These movements provided understanding, frameworks, and strategies that shaped the philosophy and tactics of Disability rights movements. 'Disability rights activists have followed the path laid by the civil rights leaders before them, seeking nothing more than equality in the eyes of society and the government' (Shapiro, 1993).

If we look at the Independent Living Movement, a movement in the US during the 1960s and 1970s which fought for the rights, autonomy, and full participation in society for Disabled people, we learn that it was significantly influenced by both the Civil Rights Movement and the Feminist Movement (Evans, 2003). Or we can look at the UK Direct Action Network (DAN), which was inspired by civil rights movements like that of the US to push for Disability rights through non-violent protests and direct action. DAN's activism was central to the advocacy for accessible transportation and other essential Disability rights.

- During the Civil Rights Movement, Black and Brown Disabled people fought for their rights.

- During the Feminist Movement, Disabled women fought for their rights.

- During the Stonewall riots, gay, lesbian, and trans people fought for their rights.

But granting rights alone does not suddenly mean a person is automatically going to be included and accepted across society. When we also consider the intersecting identities of people, protections that only target a certain group will not fully protect or include them, and as Kimberlé Crenshaw points out, these systems are interconnected, so to dismantle one we need to dismantle them all.

Forms of oppression were, and in a lot of cases still are, tools in the white man's belt to seize control and maintain power across society. Forms of oppression work together to further marginalise individuals, groups, and communities. When experiencing these overlapping forms of prejudice and discrimination, a person can feel further isolated, discriminated against, excluded, and in many cases forgotten.

Intersectionality and ableism

A woman can experience sexism while simultaneously experiencing ableism. A trans person can experience transphobia while simultaneously experiencing ableism. A Black or Brown person can experience racism while simultaneously experiencing ableism. Disability interconnects with every other piece of a person's identity, shaping their view and experiences.

While ableism is a universally shared experience for Disabled people, intersectionality helps us to understand how this can create privileges for some Disabled people, or it can further oppress others.

For example, most Disabled people have universally shared experiences of being refused, silenced, or ignored when asking for equitable support. However, a Disabled Black or Brown person might be racially profiled before getting the opportunity to even ask. While there is the mutual understanding and universal experience of not getting the support, the additional form of oppression, 'racism', has meant that the Black Disabled person has been disadvantaged – something a white Disabled person would not have had to experience, therefore benefitting them and creating a privilege because of the colour of their skin.

This privilege can be hard for a person to see or accept. But when we say you have been afforded privilege, we are not saying that you have not struggled; we are simply saying that sometimes that struggle you are experiencing is being amplified for others because of things they have no control over.

Let's look at some of the ways Disability interacts with every piece of our identity.

Disability and race and ethnicity

A Black Disabled woman will have an entirely different experience from that of a white Disabled woman or a Black Disabled trans person. While each individual will experience ableism, they will also experience other forms of oppression and for Black, Brown, Indigenous, and other people of colour, this unfortunately means racism.

Black Disabled women can experience barriers such as lower quality care, racial profiling, higher rates of maternal mortality, or being labelled with the racist 'angry Black woman' narrative. Black Disabled women often navigate the dual marginalisation of race and Disability. The 'angry Black woman' trope, when applied to Disabled women, further isolates them, as their emotional responses are dismissed, and their struggles for justice are ignored or misunderstood (Wendell, 2016).

❝ My journey as a Black, blind, and low-vision single mom, living with ADHD, is a testament to resilience within a world not always built for intersecting identities like mine. These layers of who I am – Black, Disabled, neurodivergent – aren't just labels. They are integral parts of my story that deepen my understanding of belonging, empathy, and the fight for true inclusion. Another pivotal part of this journey has been uprooting my family and moving from Houston, Texas, to Louisville, Kentucky, to take on a leadership role as Director of Inclusion, Diversity, and Equity for a century-old staple in the US.

We officially moved in March, and since then, I've encountered new challenges in integrating myself, my son, and my daughter into our new community. After just one year in the role, as a result of political oppression and massive lay-offs, I no longer occupy that role. As a Black single mom with a Disability, navigating these complex factors is mentally draining and challenges the will to persist on any given day. Beyond establishing my place professionally, I've had to ensure that my children feel safe and that they belong in their private learning institutions. As the only Black children in their classrooms, with a Disabled parent, they've faced subtle yet impactful experiences of being seen as 'different'. Our family's experience is what drives my advocacy, activism, and passion to educate, speak, and help others expand their mindsets to be compassionate and considerate of the nuanced multidimensional experience of existing in a world not designed for acceptance of who you are. 99

– Montreece Payton-Hardy, diversity, equity, and inclusion champion and change agent/inclusive leadership advisor

Being a white Disabled person brings privileges not afforded to Black, Brown, Indigenous, and other people of colour. When we add Disability to this, Black Disabled people and Disabled people who are not white face compounded discrimination. Black Disabled people in the US experience poverty at a rate of 28%, which is significantly higher than the general population rate of poverty. Hispanic Disabled people experience a poverty rate of 26% (National Disability Institute, 2019a), highlighting the additional barriers to opportunity, healthcare and support for Disabled people of colour.

Meanwhile in the UK, Disabled people, particularly from Black and ethnic minority backgrounds, face higher rates of violence and abuse, including hate crime (Disability Rights UK, 2022a). When Disability overlaps with race and ethnicity it disproportionately affects Disabled people. And within education, Disabled people from ethnic minority groups often report feeling invisible in educational content, as there is a lack of representation of both Disability and ethnicity in textbooks and teaching resources (UK Parliament, 2023a). This lack of representation isn't just about not seeing Disability represented, or race represented, but rather it is about failing to see yourself represented and failing to see the support being offered to people like you experiencing overlapping forms of oppression.

Disability and gender

Globally, 2.4 billion women of working age lack equal economic rights compared to men (World Bank, 2022). Women also report significantly higher rates of sexual violence (Smith *et al.*, 2021), and 80% of women experience street harassment based on their gender (Kearl, 2010). Men have privileges afforded to them in society that women do not, and when we consider the intersection of gender and Disability, Disabled women face compounded challenges.

A study published by *Frontiers in Psychology* found that Disabled women are frequently perceived as incapable of becoming mothers and raising children (Oswald & Penketh, 2021). Disabled women are often excluded from traditional roles associated with femininity; they are not seen as beautiful, a bride, or a mum, and so on. Society desexualises them or question their suitability to being in a relationship or being a parent. Disabled women also experience disproportionately high rates of domestic abuse compared to non-Disabled women.

According to the Office for National Statistics UK, 17.5% of Disabled women aged 16 to 59 reported experiencing domestic abuse, nearly three times the rate of non-Disabled women (Shewan Stevens, 2024). When we view this through the lens of race, socio-economic status, class, and so on, we also learn that Disabled women have the highest rates of poverty and the lowest total income levels (Maroto

& Pettinicchio, 2022). But as we know, gender is more than male and female; it includes trans and gender non-conforming people.

Transgender people, particularly transgender women of colour, face disproportionately high rates of violence. A 2013 report found that transgender people of colour were 1.5 times more likely to experience threats and intimidation, and 1.5 times more likely to experience sexual assault than white cisgender individuals (James *et al.*, 2013). Whether you are male, female, trans, non-binary, and so on, gender will impact a Disabled person's experience of ableism.

Disability and sexuality

A Disabled person's sexuality or the very idea of them being sexual and in a relationship is often ignored or overlooked: 'Who could love them?' 'They don't have sex surely, how would they even?'

LGBTQIA+ people already face significant challenges due to homophobia, lesbianphobia, biphobia, and transphobia. In a report by The Trevor Project (2024), 40% of LGBTQIA+ youth reported seriously considering suicide in the past year, as a result of social stigma, shame, inequality, and inequities. Another report from the Williams Institute (2021) shows that LGBTQIA+ individuals, especially those who are transgender, experience higher rates of unemployment and lower wages compared to their non-LGBTQ+ counterparts.

LGBTQIA+ people globally experience barriers to their rights and freedoms and in today's current climate we are watching as rights for people are rolled back, and the time to sit back and say nothing is no more. We must stand with our siblings if we are to end ableism for all Disabled people.

When we also consider that approximately 36% of LGBTQIA+ adults self-report having a Disability, compared to 24% of non-LGBTQIA+ adults (HRC Foundation, 2022), we can see that a lot of Disabled people are also LGBTQIA+. For Disabled people, especially those with non-visible Disabilities, coming out as gay, bi, trans, and so on, and then coming out as Disabled can almost feel like a double whammy. When we also consider the internalised ableism of Disabled people it should not shock you to learn that LGBTQIA+ young Disabled people report higher rates of depression, anxiety, and suicidality compared to their non-Disabled peers (The Trevor Project, 2023), extracting and creating overwhelming experience that can be difficult to articulate or understand.

Disability and geographic location

The location a Disabled person is born or resides in plays a significant role on what support is available to them. If a Disabled person is born or lives in a developed country it is more likely there are structured systems in place to support them with access to healthcare, financial support, transport infrastructure, or specialised services. For a Disabled person born or living in a developing country, their reality can be a stark contrast.

According to the World Health Organization (2022), in developing countries, more than half of Disabled people do not receive much-needed healthcare because they cannot afford the cost, and a quarter because they do not have or cannot afford transport to health facilities. This means that Disabled people will not get the medication they need, the adjustments and accommodations they need, the diagnosis they need, and the support that their Disabled peers in developed countries can access a lot more freely. For the 80% of the global Disabled population living in these developing countries (World Health Organization, 2022), this means they have not been afforded the same privileges as those born in developing countries. Now we should also add to this that even in developing countries access to healthcare or the support a person needs is not guaranteed – after all, we live in a capitalist society.

Disability and socio-economic status

The socio-economic status of a Disabled person can determine the level of opportunities and support available to a Disabled person. Socio-economic status refers to a person's position in society and includes things like their income, education level, occupation, and their access to resources. Think of a Disabled Indigenous woman from a low-income background in the US; this woman may encounter greater barriers to accessing healthcare than a white Disabled woman also in the US, but who is from a higher-income household. Although the two women will experience barriers in their everyday lives because of their Disability, one of them has a higher disposable income which creates access to resources (Wendell, 2016), whereas the Indigenous woman from a lower income background does not have the resources. The white Disabled woman has privilege; the other does not.

Disabled people face socio-economic disadvantage because of barriers to education, employment, and healthcare, leading to poverty and economic marginalisation. Research in the US indicates that across all racial and ethnic groups, 26% of Disabled individuals live below the poverty line, compared to 11% of those without Disabilities. This disparity is even more pronounced among Black and Indigenous populations with Disabilities, who experience higher poverty rates than their white counterparts (National Disability Institute, 2020).

Oppression does not exist in isolation

Now, before anyone jumps at us saying, 'Oh, but I support Disabled people; I just don't support Disabled trans people', that, my friend, is not really up for discussion. You cannot pick and choose which groups of Disabled people to support or not, as that adds to the ableism the individual will experience, which will just add other layers of oppression, transphobia, sexism, and so on.

Within the Disability space there is a saying, 'nothing about us without us'. Nothing without us means all of us, not just some of us.

We all have a responsibility to create spaces that encourage people to discuss and share all pieces of themselves. We also need to be able to represent Disability through an intersectional lens. Representing Disability in all its diversity means going beyond the white experience of Disability, going beyond just physical Disability, listening to numerous voices, and learning from diverse Disabled experiences. But what else can you do?

Within specific marginalised groups and communities, no matter how close they are, a Disabled person might struggle to open up and fully share all pieces of their identity. Instead, they opt to mask, downplay, or hide certain pieces out of fear, indifference, or sometimes due to cultural acceptance. For example, a person from a South Asian background might struggle to share that they acquired Disability with their family or friends due to cultural differences and understanding. It can feel lonely when you are unable to be your true self, when pieces of your identities are ignored or misunderstood, or when you yourself have to make the choice to hide them out of concern for your safety.

Tips for intersectional allyship

Amplify diverse Disabled voices

There is one voice that is amplified more than others, and that is the white person's experience of Disability. In panel discussions hosted online about Disability, the vast majority of these are white people talking about Disability, and while yes, some of these panellists will be Disabled themselves, it only centres one experience and does not present an accurate reflection of the Disabled experience. It is important to amplify voices of Disabled people from all diversities, and use your own power to amplify and share their work and experiences. Follow diverse Disabled content creators, advocates, trainers, and influencers online, sharing and learning from their work, and hire them if you are in a position of power.

Acknowledge the complexities of identities

As a non-Disabled person, if a Disabled person shares their experiences of Disability, you should never claim to understand what that person is going through – that is not empathy. This dismisses the very real challenges a Disabled person experiences. Yes, empathise, but do not centre yourself in their lived experience. This is also true when it comes to understanding the diverse intersectional identities that exist within the Disabled community. It is important to understand that each individual's experiences are unique to them; a person might be Disabled but they are so much more than this and that complexity cannot be ignored.

Recognise our own privilege

Everyone has privilege; even those who are oppressed will hold some form of privilege. At times, this might be hard or uncomfortable for a person to admit, but we all do, whether it is due to the colour of our skin, Disability status, gender, sex, sexuality, race, culture, and so on. We all have to realise that it is not an admission of guilt to admit privilege. It is something we all must recognise and acknowledge, if we are ever to unlearn oppression.

Stop claiming to be an expert

The word expert is thrown around the Disability space like a buzzword, as if one person can be an expert on every single Disability and the intersectional experiences that form this experience. It is important to be open to the fact that one Disabled person does not speak for a whole community. One person's experience of Disability is their experience, not everyone's experience. They are an expert on their lived experiences, not on Disability.

Be open

When you create space to talk about Disability, you have to also make space for people to share more than this piece of their identity. For example, a person might want to share their experiences of racism and ableism and how this has impacted or shaped them. But asking them to only talk about the ableism side is censoring this person's lived experience. Be open to understanding and hearing about all aspects of Disability, not just the parts you think are trendy, relevant, or on topic.

Educate yourself

We all have a responsibility to learn about the systems of oppression that exist within our society. It is privilege to believe you are exempt from needing to understand ableism, racism, sexism, and so on. This privilege is because you yourself do not experience the oppression, or you are benefitting from it. Make no mistake, you might just be contributing to systems of oppression right now, but one day you will be the one experiencing, the one disadvantaged, the one oppressed. So, start educating yourself before you start experiencing.

Represent diversity

When representing Disability, don't just show white people. Don't just show wheelchair users. Use diverse imagery to represent the intersectional experiences and identities that exist within the Disabled community. This also means not only representing Disability during Disability-specific dates (Disability Pride Month, International Day of Persons with Disabilities), but also representing Disability across the year. That includes representing Disability during LGBTQIA+ Pride Month, Black History Month, International Women's Day, and so on, and don't just represent this in your marketing. Hire Disabled speakers, consultants, and trainers across the year.

Pass the mic

Speaking for a group or community about something you don't have the lived experience of is privilege. Learning to pass the mic means allowing Disabled people to speak for themselves. This does not mean the same Disabled person speaking over and over again, but rather passing the mic to people who can speak about intersectionality. A Disabled man alone cannot lead the conversation on gender violence against Disabled girls and women; likewise white Disabled women cannot lead the conversation on racism and Disability.

Intersectionality is not a buzzword

Intersectionality is not a buzzword to be used for diversity, equity, and inclusion (DEI) initiatives, nor should it be a word Disability advocates and activists just throw around. It is about recognising things beyond our own lived experiences. It is understanding how one system which benefits us can disadvantage another. It is about respecting the diversity of experiences that exist even within one group or community. Disability and intersectionality are co-reliant conversations – you cannot discuss one without discussing the other. You cannot discuss Disability without discussing gender, race, ethnicity sex, sexual orientation, and so on.

But yet that's exactly what many organisations do. When asked about their DEI efforts they will talk about the initiatives they are doing to support ethnic hiring. Other organisations might respond with information about the work they are doing to support women in the workplace, and while all this work is vital for inclusion, we cannot disregard intersectionality. An organisation cannot focus solely on supporting racially and ethnically marginalised groups and communities without also understanding that individuals from these communities will also be Disabled, neurodivergent, straight, gay, lesbian, bi, trans, non-binary, asexual, and so on. DEI is about respecting the diversity of people, it is about creating equitable support and opportunities, and it means including everyone, not our chosen few.

This also means looking at policies through an intersectional lens, understanding that a sickness policy may impact a Disabled person differently from someone who is not Disabled. It needs to account for a woman experiencing menopause, who is Disabled, and who may need additional time off. Policies need to move beyond a one-size-should-fit-all and understand the complexities and challenges some individuals experience as a result of their intersecting identities.

Organisations that have established Disability groups/networks/employee resource groups also need to be sure they are not pigeon-holing colleagues into one group. This happens when they fail to create space and resources for colleagues who identify with multiple groups. These groups need to collaborate to facilitate conversations that go beyond one identity, to produce resources that support colleagues who face compounded disadvantages and to provide time for colleagues to be able to engage with these groups.

Diversity is not one thing. Disability is not one thing. A person's identity is not one thing. Therefore, we cannot ever hope to unlearn ableism when we are not also unlearning racism, sexism, classism, homophobia, biphobia, transphobia, and so on. Calling yourself an ally but not speaking up for LGBTQIA+ communities is not allyship. Calling yourself an ally and not challenging systemic racism or white supremacy is not allyship. Calling yourself an ally of Disabled people but disregarding and ignoring other pieces of their identities is blissful ignorance. That is not allyship, that is selective allyship, and allyship cannot be anything other than intersectional.

While writing this, we appreciate that we are both white Disabled people. We both have privileges and power as a result of this, but, as we have said, admitting your privileges is not an admission of guilt; it is the truth. We need to understand the roles we all individually play when contributing to systems of oppression, and that is what we hope you have learned from this chapter.

CHAPTER 5

Unlearning Ableism:
The History of Disability and the Disability Rights Movement

> Disabled people did not suddenly appear or arrive from another planet. We have been around since the dawn of time, a natural part of human diversity, only society didn't seem to get that memo...

Summarising Disability history in one single chapter is an unenviable task, but don't worry; luckily for you, we have done it! Buckle up because you're going to learn everything you need to know about how we got to where we are today, and how ableism became the entity it is. We must warn you, however, that this can make for an uncomfortable read. We wanted to be as honest and historically accurate as possible, but please be advised, this might make some people uncomfortable, so read at your own discretion.

> 66 History opens up exciting avenues for people to think about change over time. d/Deaf and Disabled people have likewise observed these shifts and turns, contributing to different local,

national, transnational, and global pictures. Histories of d/Deaf and Disabled people span time periods and societies, capturing not only multiple modern social and political movements, but also labour, warfare, healthcare, education, and relationships, among many other themes.

In this way, history can help link us to the past and also connect us with the present and the future. For some, this sense of knowing and reclaiming histories around rights can help to reflect on a sense of identity and belonging, both at an individual level and as part of a collective. In addition, history creates connections with activists, political organisers, and community members, both alive and those who have gone before us. From lawyers and educators to architects and artists (clearly not an exhaustive list!), d/Deaf and Disabled people have often persisted and thrived in a range of settings, albeit under sometimes hostile and oppressive conditions. With this in mind. legislation is only a small part of the historical story. While claims to rights and citizenship have long been demanded by d/Deaf and Disabled people, especially in western countries such as the UK and the US, these trajectories might not be met with a universal consensus. Histories of d/Deaf and Disabled people's rights differ considerably from country to country and are as varied as the communities themselves. 🙶

– Kirstie Stage, academic researcher

Where it all began?

Let us cast our minds right back to the very beginning. The beginning of the human species or homo sapiens, to use the fancy scientific terminology. In other words, the form of humans that we know today – think caves, fires, fight or flight, woolly mammoths, and survival of the fittest. Now the natural instinct here would be to presume that Disabled people, whether they were born Disabled or acquired their Disability, would have probably been, for want of polite language, 'kicked out' or worse. After all, back in those days hunting, foraging, and survival were what drove our mentality, and as society tells us even now, Disabled people couldn't possibly be able to contribute to such ambitions now, could they?

Well actually, think again. Scientific evidence and the excavation of ancient burial sites tells us something quite shocking. Believe it or not, how we treated Disabled people wasn't always like it was today. Archaeological evidence actually tells us that Disabled children and adults were for the most part considered equal to other members of their clans and tribes. Excavation of ancient bones of nomadic caveman in southern Italy found evidence of the care and protection for more 'vulnerable' members of their groups (Thompson *et al.*, 2025). Survival was priority number one, and that meant everyone. Archaeologists describe these findings as 'clear signs of compassion' (Kadja *et al.*, 2017).

Somewhere between our days of early homo sapiens existence to the establishment of what we now consider 'human community development', revolution and formal structures began, and so we saw the 'advancement' of our species. Here is where we start getting into a whole heap of trouble. Shift your mind from caves and fires to pillars, mythology, Romans, pyramids, and parchment.

According to the Governor's Council on Developmental Disabilities (2025), the evidence for discrimination against Disabled people and ableism within society is traceable back to the dawn of civilisation as we know it today, with biblical extracts and Roman philosophers describing the prohibition of Disabled people from marrying, having children, or integrating in society. During this time, Disability was viewed as a sign of weakness, a symbol of lack of authority, intelligence, power, and influence. Disabled children and their parents, and adults were ousted from being able to participate or contribute to society in any way. Effectively we were described as defective and a burden to civilisation. Multiple biblical and philosophical academic writings also reference illness, mental health conditions, and Disability as punishment for failure to obey religion or adhere to societal guidelines (Murphy, 2024). And well, it just got worse from here.

Moving out of caves to civilisation

As humanity began to develop and expand between the 1100s and the 1500s, so came with it outbreaks of disease, illness, and genetic conditions. With poor conditions, and a lack of medical understanding, Disabled people were in for a blooming bumpy ride. The number of children born with Disabilities rose drastically, and so did adults acquiring Disabilities. Those affected, from infant to elderly, were forcibly removed from their homes and placed into 'quarantines' with other individuals, horrifically known as 'housing for the incapacitated'. When we hear the word home we often think of a place of safety, comfort, and protection, but back in those days the dreadful conditions Disabled people were subjected to would not invoke any of these images. Disabled people were not to be seen, we were not to be heard, and were certainly not to be loved, and this was normality. They were abandoned to deteriorate in the most horrific conditions (Historic England, 2025).

Throughout the early centuries of the Common Era, any 'affliction', whether physical, neurological, or disease-borne, was viewed to be contagious. Disabled people did not know touch from others, weren't allowed to share food or even have another person enter their room. Historical documents from this time describe mothers abandoning their children in woodlands, assisted suicide, solitary confinement and murder as necessary actions. Archaeological evidence from the European leprosy outbreak between 1000 and 1400 CE only added fuel to the fire for the need for Disability segregation, meaning Disabled people were viewed to be 'failures' in the human design, the living demonstration for the need to develop and revolutionise further to prevent our existence (Historic England, 2025).

And then came the Renaissance period of the 1300s. Did it get better? Nope – this is just another walk down a dark troubled history. As people found more comfort in their existence and were no longer driven by just the primary aims of food and shelter, they wanted to be and do more (Anderson, 2020). Europe became infatuated with beauty, not just being beautiful in appearance but also the beauty in conforming to normality and through our gender-dictated roles in society. We don't think we need to explain why things were about to get a whole lot worse after learning that. Want to know something shocking? English law actually allowed and actively encouraged the discrimination of Disabled people, categorising people as either the 'deserving' and the 'undeserving' (Golightley & Holloway, 2016). It was legal and encouraged that Disabled people should not be allowed near employment, financial assets, or additional support. There was no – yes, no – state support.

Getting closer to life as we know it

In the 1500s, things must surely be getting better? Nope, not yet, hold on… With the dissolution of monasteries – entities which had previously acted as hospitals and infirmaries, providing care and support – there was a move towards caring for others being not just a religious duty but also a civic responsibility. New public-funded hospitals were built to replace the destroyed monasteries, but care and kindness were not present (Historic England, 2025).

Actually, we saw an even further regression of Disabled rights and societal perceptions. We all know the stories of the 'witches' – women who were burned and drowned for doing 'the devil's work'. What you probably don't know is an often unspoken-about truth that Disabled women of this time – those with physical, mental, and pain-inducing illnesses – were one of the greatest victims of this practice. They were hunted down and killed, and medieval doctors would perform purification rituals on the brain and skull to allow for the removal of 'evil'. The view of Disability had progressed from not only being a burden and 'unworthy' but now Disabled people were seen as having the presence of evil spirits in the soul, a living reminder to others of a religious purgatory punishment.

However, during this time the Poor Law Acts were introduced in the UK, which noted that the 'impotent poor', or more descriptively, a person who was Disabled at birth either physically or with intellectual Disabilities who couldn't work, were to be provided for (Wright, 2010). This was ambiguous in itself: 'The person naturally Disabled, either in wit or member, as an idiot, lunatic, blind, lame etc., not being able to work…all these…are to be provided for by the overseers of necessary relief and are to have allowances…according to…their maladies and needs.' We will let you guess what this meant, and whether the care received actually was 'care' (Historic England, 2025).

During the 1600s, mentality started to shift, and Disability was not seen as the consequence of God or astrological influence. Disabled people had remained in their communities as best as they could, relying on support from family and communities or sometimes assistance from wealthy local landowners – a complete pot-luck of support. Now the widely accepted view was that they belonged in institutions.

With all this going on, we know you're asking the same things too: did anybody disagree with these practices, was anybody trying to help? Historians for this point in history are only able to identify a handful of philosophers, academics, and medical professionals championing the societal reintroduction of Disabled people. To put it mildly, life for Disabled people was bleak, unbearable, and full of constant fear. Help was not forthcoming.

Here come the revolutions

We've now reached a point in history where, no pun intended, we kicked humanity up a gear. Yup, you guessed correctly, the revolutions of the 1700s. Now we're thinking about factories, metal, industry, manufacturing, and the speed of life jumping up about 1000 paces.

Urbanisation (which is basically where we made cities and towns) brought with it the introduction of asylums, workhouses, and Disability institutions. Our rights as Disabled people – well, we didn't have any. Disabled people who were previously lucky enough to remain hidden away at home were no longer able to do so; privacy as a social construct was decreasing, with an increased focus on group societal participation capabilities, living and working together equally for the good of society. You can therefore imagine that anybody who wasn't able to 'pull their weight' to the same effect was seen to be unproductive for society or the economy and needed to be removed. Those who were seen to be 'less Disabled' were put into workhouses in horrific conditions to do 'what they could'. Toddlers to the elderly, age was irrelevant. Oliver Twist isn't just a made-up story. Those who were unsuitable for these workhouses were institutionalised, subjected to horrific treatment, starved, experimented on, and abandoned. Life was now about money.

Disabled people were a burden on this mentality, treated with disrespect and contempt (Royal College of Nursing, 2025).

Jumping into the 1800s, as the revolutions slowed in the West, some of the asylums and institutions of the previous generations were renamed and rebranded as 'schools' for the 'handicapped', for Disabled people who were still being viewed as a 'threat' to our advancing society. The institutionalisation of Disabled people was for life; children were sent never to return to their families, subjected to horrific treatments, experiments, and unacceptable care. The institutionalisation of Disabled people at this time was predominately used for those with 'visible Disabilities', as those with non-visible, mental health, and chronic conditions were typically unable to survive the awful living conditions or deemed not 'Disabled enough' to be taken away (The Open University, 2025).

By 1900, over 100,000 Disabled people, referred to as 'idiots and lunatics', had been removed from their communities to 'pauper asylums'. In the early 1900s, as education and medical practices began to be prioritised, there was an increased focus on the 'mental deficiencies' and 'insanity' of those who were 'morally defect'. Being able to 'contribute' to society didn't just mean physical contribution any more. This meant that more and more of those with mental health conditions and neurological conditions were sent away to institutions (Jarret, 2023).

Surely, as there were massive gains in understanding, education, and medicine, the perception of Disability must have been shifting, even if slightly, in the right direction? Nope. Despite a few medical professionals and academics campaigning for better treatment, there was little to no progress. Disabled people were isolated, prevented from participation, unable to marry, and hidden away. Medical experimentation, sterilisation, and the use of patients as specimens were normal practices.

Eugenics

Eugenics is a painful historical lesson on how intersecting identities, such as being Disabled and poor, Disabled and a woman, or Disabled and a person of colour can be used to further marginalise and dehumanise Disabled people. But what exactly is eugenics?

Eugenics is a set of beliefs and practices that sets out to improve the genetic quality of a population by controlling who is allowed to reproduce. This was achieved by ensuring people who were deemed to have undesirable characteristics and traits based on race, Disability, gender, class, or socio-economic status could not reproduce and by placing restrictions on them. Historically, it has been used as a pseudoscientific justification for discrimination, forced sterilisation, and even genocide (Uldry & EDF Women's Committee, 2022).

During the eugenics movement in the 20th century, people of colour, immigrants, and Disabled people were labelled and viewed as morally defective. Eugenicists believed that by controlling human reproduction they could enhance the human race with what they perceived to be 'desirable traits'. Sound familiar? It should. Eugenics played a significant role in the Second World War. During this time, the Nazi eugenics campaign systematically murdered millions of Jews, as well as Disabled people, gay men, and other categories of people that were deemed to be inferior. During this time, the Aktion T4 euthanasia program (1939–1945) led to the systematic murder of 200,000 Disabled individuals in Germany and Austria (Friedlander, 1995).

But it was not just Nazi Germany where the ideology of eugenics was embraced. Other countries in the world such as the US, Canada, and parts of Europe used this as a lawful way to justify forced sterilisation. Between the 1920s and the 1940s it is estimated that 40–50% of all sterilisation victims in the US were people labelled as Disabled, particularly those deemed 'mentally ill,' 'feeble-minded,' or 'epileptic', and a disproportionate number of Disabled women were sterilised; in many cases, they were institutionalised specifically to be sterilised (Stern, 2005). And in Sweden between 1934 and 1976, about 63,000 sterilisations occurred, with many targeting Disabled people under the pretence of preventing 'inferior' traits from being passed on (Broberg & Tydén, 2005).

But it wasn't just forced sterilisation or institutionalisation that individuals experienced; there were restrictions on relationships and marriages, and policies that sought to dehumanise and ostracise these people. In many cases, if a Disabled person was already married but deemed 'genetically unfit', they were often subjected to forced divorce and sterilisation (Friedlander, 1995).

People of colour, immigrants, Jewish people, Disabled people, and LGBTQIA+ people suffered at the expense of the eugenics movement. It is a painful lesson on how systems of oppression don't just co-exist but rather they prop up and reinforce each other, often justifying the others' cause and providing new ways to further control and oppress.

The legacy of the eugenics movement is evident in the historical overuse of institutionalisation, the stigmatisation of Disability, and ongoing debates about reproductive rights and genetic testing.

We wish we could say that the forced sterilisation of Disabled people now doesn't happen in the world, but this would be a lie. In a 2022 report by the European Disability Forum, 13 countries across Europe had legal frameworks permitting guardians, legal representatives, or medical professionals to authorise sterilisation procedures on behalf of Disabled people, often without their explicit consent (Uldry & EDF Women's Committee, 2022). The 13 countries identified were:

- Bulgaria
- Croatia
- Cyprus
- Czechia
- Denmark
- Estonia
- Finland
- Hungary
- Latvia
- Lithuania
- Malta
- Portugal
- Slovakia.

In 2024, campaigners increased efforts to implement a European Union-wide ban on forced sterilisation across member states, but despite these efforts, as of early 2025 legislation prohibiting this practice across all member states has not yet been enacted (Demony, 2024).

And these nations are not alone. In countries like China, India, Indonesia, Mexico, Peru, Brazil, and South Africa, forced sterilisation remains an active threat to Disabled people, particularly Disabled women.

Eugenics may not be as glaringly obvious today, but it is evidenced in society's need to label things as 'normal', 'fit', and 'healthy'. It is evidenced in the institutionalised racism, sexism, ableism, and so on that still exists today. It is present in prenatal screenings, where testing can identify Disabilities within a foetus, and it can be found in gene editing. In the UK, approximately 90% of pregnancies diagnosed with Down syndrome through prenatal testing end in selective abortion (Office for Health Improvement & Disparities, 2022). Gene editing has the potential to edit out genetic conditions, raising the question, what constitutes a desirable life?

We are not here to answer this but rather we make the point that while this is not a direct application of eugenics, the high rate of abortion based on genetic conditions raises ethical concerns about modern-day 'genetic selection' and its potential eugenic undertone.

This was a contributing factor to the Second World War and after the collapse of the Nazi regime in Europe, eugenics took a bit of a back seat, but is always there.

World wars

The First and Second World Wars of the 1900s brought mass devastation around the world and initiated a turning of the tide for Disability. For the first time, we acquired protection by law and a degree of social movement. But at great cost. Injured and unwell servicemen and women returning from the war were greeted with care and attention from grateful nations across the world, and for almost the first time, medical and social provisions were rolled out, not banishment or ostracisation. Disabled people were shown care, attention, love, rehabilitation, and proper facilities (Maloney, 2017).

However, we did tell you it was only a smidge of a corner – those who were not injured or ill servicemen and women, but Disabled people who had not partaken in the 'war effort', still faced institutionalisation. Despite a mild improvement in perceptions and attitudes towards Disabled people, stereotyping and the misconception of Disabilities prevailed, with the use of asylums and institutions still rife. Disabled people were often left to die, left in pain, and subjected to horrendous treatment. Those who were not deemed 'Disabled enough' for institutions struggled with any additional support, were ignored in their communities, and hidden away (Historic England, 2025).

As we moved further into the 1900s, something quite incredible happened. In the 1940s, we had one of our first moments of victory for the Disability Rights Movement – the introduction of the Disability Employment Act, and Disability-related health initiatives. The pace of Disabled rights progression got its kick (Barnes & Mercer, 2004). And there was a further kick in the UK.

In 1948, the National Health Service (NHS) was introduced. Disabled people and their families, previously removed from society, had better access to medicine, treatments, and support (NHS England, n.d.). Not only this, but now medical information was more publicly available, families of Disabled children, partners of Disabled adults, teachers, nurses, and organisations all had better awareness and understanding.

The introduction of the welfare state also brought previously unseen social and financial protections. It turns out 1948 was a pretty big year for us Disabled folk, as it also brought with it the first ever Paralympic Games! For one of the first times in history, the talent, potential, and participation of Disabled people were highlighted and celebrated by the masses (International Paralympic Committee, 2025). And in America came the establishment of the National Federation of the Blind in 1940. The fear surrounding Disability decreased, and it was no longer mass associated with contagion, evilness, and punishment. By the end of the 1940s, the health disparity gap was reducing, but stereotyping and the perceptions of Disabled people as a burden on society had begun to rise with the introduction of additional taxation to provide welfare support.

By the 1970s and 1980s, the Social Model of Disability was brought into the spotlight (an important bit of information to understand in our journey to unlearn ableism – head to Chapter 1 to learn more after you've finished up here!) (Sense, n.d.). And we had some pretty big wins such as the Rehabilitation Act of 1973 in the US and the founding of the American Coalition of Citizens with Disabilities (ACCD) in 1975 (Temple University Institute on Disabilities, n.d.). This social movement of Disability played a huge role in the abolition of institutions and asylums, with the Jay Report highlighting the need for care in the community. Care in the community, not just as a nation, started to play a bigger and bigger role, with local provisions and more accessibility community support. Since the 1980s we have seen the introduction of a number of important pieces of legislation for the protection of Disabled people's rights (more details to be found in Chapter 8 on legislation and policies), and the adoption of international legislation. Yay! We are finally making progress (Mitchell, 2003).

America founded the Americans with Disabilities Act in 1990, which inspired the world, and so came the UK Disability Discrimination Act five years later (Meldon, 2015). For one of the first times both Disabled and non-Disabled people engaged together publicly in campaigning for better protections, highlighting the importance of care, accessibility, and equality.

Modern-day Disability activism

Because of the incredible work of our predecessors, we have a whole ream of celebrations and achievements to be proud of, markers of how far we have come. To name but a few:

- **Purple Tuesday:** Founded in 2018, an annual event dedicated to promoting accessibility and inclusivity for Disabled consumers, serving as a reminder of the importance of making businesses and public spaces more accessible to individuals with Disabilities, including physical, sensory, and cognitive impairments. The event encourages organisations to take steps towards improving their accessibility and ensuring that Disabled customers can enjoy equal access to products, services, and experiences.

- **Disability Pride Month:** Celebrated every year in July since 1990 following the creation of the Americans with Disabilities Act and the Boston Disability marches (BBC Newsround, 2023).

- **World Mental Health Day:** An annual global day since 1992 of education, awareness, and advocacy, opposing the social stigmas of mental health.

- **Global Accessibility Awareness Day:** Launched in 2012, this focuses on digital access and inclusion for all Disabled people around the world with the purpose to get everyone talking, thinking, and learning about digital (web, software, mobile, etc.) access or inclusion and people with different Disabilities.

- **And so many others, such as:** World Braille Day, Carer's Week, Learning Disability Week, World Sight Day, Neurodiversity Celebration Week. There are too many to mention without filling the whole chapter (Business Disability Forum, 2025)! All of these days, weeks, and months hold such incredible value as tools to promote education, awareness, and access for Disabled people across the world. So, whether you are an organisation, a Disabled individual, or an ally, find out how you can be celebrating Disability and advocating for yourself or other Disabled people in your journey of unlearning ableism.

Now, you may have noticed something pretty major missing from this list. Drum roll please…hello United Nations and the Convention and International Day of Persons with Disabilities. Now we are going to explore the Convention itself more in our legislation and policies chapter; it is a result of decades of fighting by Disability advocates for better international legal protections for Disabled people. In 1981, the United Nations held the first ever International Year of Disabled Persons, and then between 1983 and 1992 there was 'The Decade of Disabled Persons'! Although we would all like another decade, every year we have celebrated International Day on 3 December since 1992. It is arguably the biggest celebration of Disability each year (did you know that the Convention was one of the quickest ever supported human rights instruments in history?) (Inclusion Canada, n.d.).

Something we also have now, that we most definitely didn't before, are our widely accepted and used metaphors and narratives championed by the Disabled community to educate and create awareness. For example, as mentioned earlier in the book, 'nothing about us without us' and 'spoon theory', coined in 2003 by Christine Miserandino to describe physical and mental energy expenditure and explain barriers for non-Disabled people.

The power of social media

And we cannot ignore the power of social media and the influence this has had on the Disability Rights Movement. Social media has become a powerful tool for the Disability community and for advancing Disability rights. Its impact has built community, generated advocacy and activism, shared resources, support, and information, created space for the amplification of previously unheard voices, highlighted accessibility, influenced policy and law, provided resources for education and training, and fostered innovation led by the Disabled community. Social media has created a space for empowerment, facilitating communication, advocacy, and education.

It provides a platform for individuals to share their experiences, connect with others, and push for change, ultimately fostering greater awareness and understanding of Disability rights and issues. However, it is important to acknowledge the digital divide and ensure that everyone, regardless of their circumstances, has access to these platforms.

All of these key moments in our Disability history have been instrumental in raising awareness, challenging discrimination, and promoting the rights and inclusion of individuals with Disabilities. They have paved the way for greater recognition, protection, and advancement of Disability rights and have inspired continuing efforts to build a more inclusive and equitable society for all.

We want to take a moment at this point of our unlearning journey to acknowledge the incredible campaigners from across our history who dedicated their lives to the Disability Rights Movement. We would not be where we are now without your passion and commitment. For all the generations to come, we thank you. We also want to take a moment to remember those who lost their lives throughout history as a result of the despicable treatment of Disabled people, those who lost their lives unnecessarily, those who suffered and experienced such pain and hardship. You will never be forgotten.

So, where are we now?

In the last 30 or so years, for Disabled people we have seen better access to medical support, more laws that protect us, more campaigns, more charities, more governing bodies, better accessibility, better care and better equity. But – this is a big but – although we have come a long way from institutions, asylums, and abhorrent medical practices, with communal recognition of the abominable previous treatments of Disabled people, we are actually only very near the beginning of the mass journey in Disability rights. Is it better? Absolutely. Is it perfect? Definitely not.

66 Whether it fills you with discomfort, a sense of pride, or is simply a descriptor, 'Disability' has carried a weight far heavier than its syllables suggest. Disabled people have always existed. But history has often chosen to define us rather than allow us to define ourselves. Language reflects power, and the way Disability has been framed over centuries – from medieval religious narratives of sin and suffering to today's debates over economic 'burdens' – has shaped how society sees us, and how we see ourselves. The word 'Disability' itself entered the English language in 1545, a by-product of a society increasingly obsessed with categorisation. Yet, long before words like 'Disability' existed, Disabled people were part of communities, contributing, loved and loving, resisting, surviving. Rights, however, have never been freely given; they have been fought for. Legislative milestones like the Disability Discrimination Act (1992) in the UK or the Americans with Disabilities Act (1990) in the US were not gifts from benevolent governments but hard-won victories by Disabled activists. Still, legal protections are only as strong as the cultures that uphold them. Disability history is not one history; it is many. And it is global. In some cultures, Disabled people are revered; in others, erased. Global approaches often fail by imposing 'universal' solutions without considering local context. If we want true change, we must recognise that Disability rights are human rights, that inclusion cannot be an afterthought, and that the stories we tell today will shape the world Disabled people inherit tomorrow. 99

– Rachael Mole CF, accessibility consultant, writer, and public speaker

The history of Disability rights is incredibly complex and ever-evolving and while it has made progress over time, the misconceptions, inaccessibility, and inequalities faced by Disabled people have been around since the dawn of civilisation as we know it.

Ableism is institutionalised into the very systems that govern our worlds, and built into the foundations of our world as we know it today. It is quite literally part of the human psyche; our whole social development over thousands of years has been built on an incorrect ideology of Disability, and one that is going to take much more time to tear apart and unlearn. The need to be proactive and not reactive is one that cannot be over-emphasised enough. Despite our advancements, challenges and barriers for Disabled people persist, including ongoing discrimination, lack of accessibility, and limited opportunities for full inclusion. We cannot just clip back the branches; we have to remove the problem from the root.

It is important that we remember that Disability rights, access to spaces, and societal perceptions vary from place to place. Not everyone shares the same privileges, and we are all at different points in our journey. Each place has its own history, influences, and journey taken and to be taken. This is due to multiple factors such as political will, economic resources, international influence, conflict, legal frameworks, cultural shifts, industrialisation, and international membership. The differences in Disability rights across countries are shaped by a complex interplay of cultural, legal, political, economic, historical, and social factors. Addressing these disparities often requires a multifaceted approach that considers the unique context of each country, remembering that we all hold the power to influence others.

CHAPTER 6

Unlearning Ableism:
Disabled by Society

> **Navigating a society not designed for you is a bit like trying to do yoga in a phone booth – awkward, uncomfortable, and you'll probably end up needing help to get out.**

Okay, so we are not encouraging you to climb inside a phone box to test out what it's like to navigate a Disabling society – please do not try this at home.

Disabled people are not treated as equals across society. We are not thought of as successful, fashionable, independent, or that we could be lovers, parents, athletes, or heaven forbid, employed or have founded a business! Instead, we are:

- excluded, overlooked or treated with pity
- forgotten in design
- left out of decision making
- not represented
- applauded for doing the bare minimum
- expected to just smile and overcome.

Most people see or learn of our Disability and assume incompetence.

Assume unintelligence. Assume not capable. Being Disabled by society is like trying to solve a Rubik's cube, except every time you manage to line up one piece, something comes along and scrambles it again.

- We ask for representation, and they give us a token character with no depth.
- We ask for accessibility, and they tell us it's too expensive.
- We ask to be included, and we're labelled woke.

No matter how much progress we make, at times it can feel as if society keeps shifting the goalposts. We get over one barrier but find ourselves encountering yet another.

> " Growing up as a wheelchair user has always thrown challenges in front of me, and I normally overcome them. However, one of the hardest challenges has been dealing with the assumptions about what I can and cannot do. These assumptions can range from underestimating my capabilities to over-generalising my needs based on other wheelchair users. One common misconception is that people with Disabilities are inherently less capable, less ambitious, and take more time off work. This couldn't be further from the truth!
>
> For instance, I remember a time when I was applying for a job at a local grocery store when I was coming out of college, and it required basic skills that I felt I could meet, such as good customer service. Despite my will and determination, I felt the interviewer seemed unable to look past my wheelchair. This assumption not only undermined my abilities, but also highlighted a broader issue: the tendency to view any Disability through a narrow lens instead of asking questions to understand our capabilities.

Another assumption I've faced is the belief that people with Disabilities are always in need of help. While support is important, it's crucial to recognise that many of us strive for independence and autonomy. I recall an incident where a stranger insisted on helping me place my wheelchair into my vehicle, despite my polite refusals. This well-intentioned gesture, though appreciated, stemmed from the assumption that I couldn't manage on my own. 〟

– Mohammad Koheeallee, accessibility, safety, health, and environment consultant

Cultural differences and treatment of Disabled people

Culturally, the way Disabled people are treated varies across the world. What's considered normal or socially acceptable in one culture might be viewed as rude or disrespectful in another. These cultural differences may not be known to an outsider or visitor, which can make travelling as a Disabled person difficult. This can also impact the way we speak or communicate with others about Disability.

For example, in the UK people lean towards identity first language: 'Disabled person'. However, in Russia, the term 'инвалид' is still commonly used in official and everyday language, but it has negative connotations, as it translates as inability or worthlessness. If you were to use this language in the UK or in other parts of western society, this would be disrespectful or unacceptable.

❝ As a public speaker, consultant, and content creator on Disability, I find that ableism shows up in both my personal and my work life. I was born in the US but have been to almost 40 countries, travelling full time for the past five years. I'm deafblind due to Usher syndrome. When I share online about my exciting travel adventures, I receive comments questioning why I even travel if I can't see or hear (most people don't know that both vision and hearing are spectrums, so I do hear and see a bit). The idea that travel isn't worthwhile without vision or hearing is an ableist one.

When I travel around the world, I use a white cane. My hearing Disability is not usually apparent to others, even though I wear hearing aids. Many countries don't have independent blind people out and about due to a lack of accessibility, but people seem to assume it's because of blind people and some incapacity we have instead. This is ableism.

People think I can't be independent due to my blindness. In Medellin, Colombia, a man gave me a teddy bear sticker, which he said he usually gives to kids, for apparently being Disabled and outside, which is not any special feat, but he seemed to feel it was. This was also infantilising because I'm not a child. In Porto, Portugal, a man grabbed my arm when I was waiting to cross the street in a group of people. It was jarring and disconcerting. He was agitated and seemed to think I needed help. I gave no signs of needing help, and I was upset to have a stranger touching my body.

Disabled people don't always need help. That's another ableist assumption. When I'm navigating independently, I want to have autonomy. Sometimes I get lost, but then it's up to me to decide if I want to ask for help or if I want to take extra time and figure it out on my own. That's part of my autonomy and dignity, and the people around me should respect that. 99

– Catarina Rivera, MSEd, MPH, CPACC, public speaker and consultant at Blindish Latina LLC

Of course, some cultures are more accepting and supportive of Disability, while others can be rejecting or isolating. Some cultures link Disability to religious or supernatural beliefs, often framing Disabled people as cursed, sinful, or divinely chosen, while some Indigenous cultures view Disability as a form of spiritual insight rather than a deficit.

Let's look at other some other cultural disparities with Disability.

Self-identifying

- In countries like the US, UK, Canada, Australia, and parts of Europe, large portions of Disabled people engage in self-advocacy and discuss their Disabilities openly to raise awareness and fight for rights.

- In Japan and some other Asian cultures, Disability isn't always openly discussed, and families might feel shame or embarrassment, typically avoiding public conversations about the Disabled family member.

- In Middle Eastern and some African cultures, Disability can be viewed as a private or family matter and openly talking about it could be seen as disrespectful or inappropriate.

Stigma

- In western cultures, Disability rights movements push for the idea that society disables people, not their impairments, which at times proves challenging as we are challenging a society that has deep rooted itself in the medical model of Disability.

- In India and some African countries, there are communities which believe that Disability is the result of karma, ancestral sins, or curses.

- In China and some east Asian cultures, Disability is sometimes viewed as shameful, which in turn brings shame to the family.

Media perception

- In western media (Hollywood, UK TV, etc.), we are seeing an increase of Disability visibility, although often portrayed inspirationally or tragically.

- In Bollywood and other Asian film industries, Disabled characters are often shown as objects of pity or for comic relief.

- In Scandinavian countries, representation focuses more on inclusion and normalisation, portraying Disabled people as equal members of society rather than as inspiration or tragedy.

Assisted mobility

- In the US, UK, and western Europe, there tends to be more access with ramps, lifts, and accessible transport available (though still with barriers, might we add).

- In Japan and South Korea, many wheelchair users experience extreme difficulty with accessibility, and there is a cultural expectation that family members will assist and care for them rather than demanding public accessibility.

- In some parts of Africa and rural Asia, wheelchair users can face social exclusion or even being hidden away by families due to stigma. In some communities, there's limited understanding of Disability beyond a medical or superstitious perspective.

Guide dogs and service animals

- In the US, UK, and Canada, guide dogs and service animals are legally protected and allowed in most public places, including restaurants and on transport, although this is not always the case as many Disabled people with service animals can attest to.

- In the Middle East and some Asian countries, many places ban dogs indoors for religious or cultural reasons, which can make it difficult for blind people to navigate public spaces.

- In Japan and South Korea, while guide dogs are legally allowed, public awareness is low, and some businesses still refuse entry to Disabled people with service animals.

> ❝ I was born in an urban slum where survival wasn't a given, where dyslexia, dyspraxia, and a stammer weren't quirks but barriers to being taken seriously. Where caregiving wasn't a noble sacrifice but a brutal, unpaid necessity because my chronically ill mother had nowhere else to turn. My body, my brain – none of it ever fitted into the clean, able-bodied lines society expected. But here's the thing: I don't need fixing. The world does. The idea that we, the Disabled, must bend ourselves to an inaccessible, indifferent society is an outdated, ableist lie. Inclusion isn't about making space at the table – it's about tearing the damn table apart and rebuilding it with all of us in mind.

> And then, climate change entered the equation. The brutal summer of 2022 in Delhi was a wake-up call. The heatwave, thick with pollution, made my stammer worse, my dyspraxia harder to navigate, my dyslexia more exhausting. It wasn't just uncomfortable; it was disabling in ways I hadn't fully grasped before. When I started speaking with others – wheelchair users

stuck in inaccessible disaster shelters, blind individuals left behind in evacuations, people with chronic illnesses unable to survive power outages – it became painfully clear. Disabled people are disproportionately affected by climate change, yet we are completely absent from its discourse. We aren't in the planning meetings, the policy rooms, or the so-called 'inclusive' sustainability conversations. That's why I started Green Disability – because we refuse to be invisible when the planet itself is turning against us.

Ableism is not just a lack of ramps, captions, or workplace accommodations. It's systemic neglect, the collective shrug that says, 'This is just how things are.' It's watching people pity a Disabled child in school but not funding their education. It's celebrating an autistic employee's 'resilience' while refusing to implement flexible working hours. It's the false narrative that our needs are expensive, burdensome, and optional. People argue that accessibility is costly, but so is exclusion. How many minds, how much talent, how many brilliant Disabled people are being shut out because society refuses to redesign itself? And let's not even start on the medical model of Disability, which treats our existence as a problem rather than confronting the actual problem: a world unwilling to adapt. Climate change, ableism, inaccessibility – these are not separate issues. They are interconnected crises that demand intersectional solutions. And we, the Disabled community, are ready to lead that fight. 99

– Puneet Singh Singhal, Co-founder of Billion Strong

Moving back to what we discussed in our intersectionality chapter, where a Disabled person is born or lives plays a fundamental role in their access to support, healthcare, education, and so on.

Disabled culture

Disabled culture is rich and filled with diverse perspectives, just like any other culture in our society, each individual with their own unique set of beliefs, views, and values, which connects them to others. Here are some examples of subcultures:

- **Neurodiversity:** This movement, driven by neurodivergent communities, promotes the idea that neurological differences should be accepted and respected rather than pathologised.

- **Crip culture:** Some Disabled people reclaim the term 'crip' as a form of empowerment, using it to challenge stereotypes and redefine what it means to live with a Disability.

- **Chronic illness communities:** Those with chronic illnesses, such as fibromyalgia, multiple sclerosis, or chronic fatigue syndrome, often build their own networks and develop their own culture, characterised by shared experiences of living with invisible Disabilities.

There is no one Disabled community; there are communities within communities, with their own cultures, beliefs, and views of the world. We're not saying we are all enemies but also we are not sitting around a campfire singing 'Kumbaya'. Being Disabled does not necessarily mean you agree with the Disabled individuals sitting next to you, or the Disabled person who has the same condition as you.

Think of a person who is d/Deaf. People will automatically group these individuals together, naively thinking they are part of the d/Deaf community, when actually within this community there are subcultures and communities with diverse lived experiences and beliefs.

Sign language is not universal. British Sign Language is not the same as American Sign Language or other sign languages around the world. The signs and expressions used within different sign languages create distinct communities.

There are also d/Deaf people who use a cochlear implant, a medical device that can provide a sense of sound to some people, and those who believe it is an attack on Deaf culture.

There are d/Deaf people who can hear or speak and there are those who cannot. d/Deaf people also have their own Deaf Pride, celebrating Deaf culture, advocating for full access to sign language, interpreting services, and education.

There are subcultures created within this one community, creating lots of communities and groups, not just for d/Deaf people but across the many diverse communities that exist across Disability.

Being Disabled by society, while we are trying to manage ableism, while also juggling ableism, is like spinning plates, throwing frisbees all while doing the Macarena. It is exhausting!

Throughout this book you will learn just how much society disables and how much everything is interconnected through ableism – and why one chapter alone is not enough to convey this!

CHAPTER 7
Unlearning Ableism: Language

> 'You can't use that word.' 'Disabled is a negative word.' 'It's person first language.' 'No, it's identity first language.' 'We should be saying differently abled.' 'Everyone is a little bit autistic.' 'Everyone just needs to calm down and stop playing top trumps with language.'

Before we talk about ableism and language, we need to say that language is complex. The historical context and meaning of words should always be respected; however, it is also important to recognise the evolution of language. Words which were once acceptable may not be tomorrow, and words that were previously avoided are now being reclaimed. We also cannot discuss language without understanding the variations in language across regions. For example, in the US we tend to see person first language used when discussing Disability ('person with Disability'), whereas in the UK it is a lot more common to come across identity first language ('Disabled person'). If we look at parts of Europe, the term 'handicap' is used by people with lived experience, whereas in the UK this term would be heavily considered ableist. And as we said in the previous chapter, in Russia the term 'инвалид', although used in official and everyday language, has negative connotations, as it translates as inability or worthlessness. If this language was used in the UK or in other parts of western society, it would be seen as disrespectful and unacceptable.

So, when we are talking about language and Disability, we have to do so with the knowledge that language evolves, and it is not universally the same in every part of the world. Respect regional-specific language, respect the voice of lived experience, and, most importantly, be open to the fact that what you consider might be ableist, might just be empowering for another.

> 66 In our global society, ableism manifests not only in overt discrimination but also in the subtle narratives that shape our cultural lens. Each community – steeped in unique traditions, religious teachings, and historical contexts – frames Disability in its own light. What one society may see as a challenge, another might revere as a distinct strength. Unlearning ableism starts with acknowledging these diverse interpretations and questioning the norms that confine our perceptions. It calls for us to dismantle outdated ideologies that value individuals solely based on conventional standards of ability.
>
> Language, in this transformation, becomes both a tool and a battleground. Our words have historically boxed people into roles, limiting their opportunities and silencing their voices. By consciously choosing inclusive language and crafting new narratives, we can celebrate the multifaceted contributions of Disabled individuals. Empowerment lies in making room for these voices – voices that bring insights not only about personal resilience but also about innovative ways of engaging with the world.
>
> Furthermore, recognising the intersectionality of Disability with culture, race, and socioeconomic status deepens our

understanding of the systemic barriers at play. When we empower individuals from varied backgrounds to share their stories, we spark a collective reimagining of what it means to be capable. Through this process, we learn to value different perspectives, breaking free from the narrow definitions imposed by tradition. In this evolving dialogue, Disability transforms from a label of limitation into a testament to human diversity and strength. "

– Tumi Sotire, The Black Dyspraxic

We are unaware

When discussing Disability, a person can either intentionally or unintentionally perpetrate harm on a person or a community. Words evoke emotions, they evoke reactions, so when talking about a person's lived experiences or the barriers they face, we must do so with sensitivity. Say the wrong thing and you might inadvertently dismiss the very real struggles of this person. Say the right thing and you could be the reason this person smiles that day or feels safe to self-identify in the future. But if you choose to correct the language a person uses to self-identify, you may unknowingly send that person spiralling with their internalised ableism.

Most people are completely unaware of the ableism ingrained in their language. They are unaware of the emotional and physical harm their language has caused, nor do they always see the pain on a person's face when they are subjected to ableism, when they are forced to listen to words that they've only ever experienced as weapons. It can be hard to understand the harm you push onto others when you say the ableist wrong thing. In these moments, you are oblivious to the ripples of your actions, but to a Disabled person, it is quite clear that Disabled people are less than, that they are the problem, that they are inferior. You remind them that to be Disabled is a negative bad thing.

The harsh reality of this is that for Disabled people, it is important to be open to the fact that people are going to make mistakes. We know it will happen. It happens now. It happens frequently. So as much as ableist language is harmful, it is also something we have had to live with.

Research by Leonard Cheshire (2022) revealed that 52% of Disabled workers reported experiencing ableist language in the workplace, contributing to exclusion and lower promotion rates. A study by the Anti-Bullying Alliance (2019) found that children who experience ableist language at school were more likely to struggle with self-esteem and academic performance (Anti-Bullying Alliance, 2019). Ableist language leaves its mark. The Mental Health Foundation (2021) reported that exposure to demeaning or ableist language significantly increases anxiety and depression among Disabled individuals.

What language *should* I be using?

There's an ongoing debate about which language a person should use when talking about Disabled people/people with Disabilities. It is a tale as old as time. 'Disabled person is better.' 'No, person with Disability is better.' It's like a never-ending game of table tennis, only there is no winner.

People spend so long going back and forth on what is right and what is wrong to say, that it has allowed ableist euphemisms to appear in these words' stead. 'Differently abled', 'different abilities', 'special', 'enabled', 'handicapable', 'unique abilities'. These words and phrases manifested because people feared saying Disabled person or person with Disability. This is a fear that the Disabled community have helped create themselves.

This debate has caused fear, as the debate is not always between Disabled and non-Disabled people. The debate happens between Disabled people and people with Disabilities. Between Disabled people and parents of children with Disabilities. Between parents of Disabled children and parents of children with Disabilities.

Throughout the ages, Disability was a source of fear, a negative, dirty thing to be ashamed of and stay clear of. The language used to define Disability during this time only sought to further divide and demonise. People opted for words instead like 'cripple', 'lame', 'deformed', 'feeble-minded', 'moron', 'imbecilic', 'handicapped'. Words that belittled. Words that degraded. Words that sought to divide. Words that made it easier to cast us aside, lock us away. Words that evoked fear or disgust. Words that sadly surface in our present day.

Today, people tend to shy away from using Disabled and Disability believing them to be negative, and instead opting for fluffy language which they feel is more positive. This language only seeks to make non-Disabled people feel more comfortable, completely unaware that these sugar-coated euphemisms are actually reinforcing the ableist lie, that to say Disabled and Disability is bad. Sadly, ableist euphemisms have become a way for a person to indirectly mention Disability, without having to use the dreaded D word. These euphemisms only seek to make the user feel more comfortable. They do not seek to comfort a Disabled person; what they do is shape the view that we shouldn't be talking about Disability or being Disabled, that they are shameful words or dirty words.

These euphemisms are created by non-Disabled people who

have good intentions but sadly do not listen to the voices of lived experiences – people in positions of power, teachers, educators, doctors; people who do not have the lived experience but lead the conversation. As we know by now, you cannot speak for a whole community, especially if you do not have the lived experience of that community.

So, let's dissect some of the more commonly used euphemisms.

Differently abled

This term came to light during the 1980s, as a way for people to avoid saying presumed negative words like Disabled. It causes problems because it completely neglects the ableist and inaccessible barriers a Disabled person experiences. It implies that to be Disabled is to be different, and not a good kind of difference. It creates a comparison between non-Disabled people and Disabled people while reinforcing the outdated belief we should not say Disabled or Disability. We should note that in parts of Asia, the term differently abled has been adopted by people with lived experiences, and the term Disabled is considered negative – regional and cultural relationships with language should always be considered.

Special

The word special has long been used within education and care settings to label Disabled people. It was a way in the 20th century to describe children with Disabilities, and adults in care settings. Special is still used commonly today; we have terms like 'special needs' and 'special education' to describe education that has been adapted for Disabled people. Due to this, the word special is often given young Disabled people who then grow up with an enforced label and way of being identified. Most of us learn, however, that being special is not a good thing. Special is a way to be labelled as different; a way for others to talk to you as though you do not understand.

Adults use the word special as though being Disabled means we get special treatment. In reality, of course, special means to be treated differently, as less than, in a society where special is not so special. Many Disabled advocates and activists advise against this language and we absolutely stand by this. This patronising label doesn't just stay with us just during childhood – as adults we face the same patronising tone of non-Disabled people telling us how special we are. They may feel safer using a word that completely overlooks and dismisses the very challenges of Disabled people, the very real barriers we face, and the very real exclusion we experience as a result.

Special has often meant segregation. Within education, young Disabled people have historically been segregated into special needs classes or into special education because mainstream education has not been designed to be accessible. It was created to support a one-size-fits-all learning. It is not accessible. Educators are not aware of how to provide equitable support and in a lot of cases, classes are so bursting with pupils that teachers simply do not have the resources to provide equitable learning. And so young Disabled people are segregated into these special classes or schools, limiting their interaction with non-Disabled peers, and often at times feeling isolated.

We also have to face a harsh truth. Kids can be mean, and within the education sector, the term special has been used as a way for non-Disabled kids to identify those who are different and in doing so providing a justification to exclude, insult, or bully them. The term special carries trauma for a lot of Disabled people. We need to transition away from labelling Disabled people as special, and labelling their needs as special, because all it does is undermine and play down a person's lived experiences.

Being Disabled does not make us special. Our needs are not special.

We have access needs. We have accessibility needs. We may require adjustments and accommodations. But that does not make us special. It means we navigate things in a way that is comfortable and accessible for us. Besides, if being Disabled was so special, surely society would be designed for us? Shocker that it is not. Special is code for, 'Aww, a poor Disabled person'. Special assumes. Special disables. Special carries trauma. Let's please unlearn it.

Additional needs

Much like the term special needs, additional needs imply that being Disabled means we have additional needs. Shocker, everyone has needs, not just Disabled people. Even bigger shocker, not every Disabled person has access needs. See what we did there? We used the word access needs, because that is what should be said, rather than making Disabled people's needs over the top, more, or additional. We all have needs. Needs can change depending on circumstances, but there is no necessity to suddenly start labelling anyone with a new need as having additional needs. So why is it done for Disabled people's needs?

It should not surprise you to learn that the term additional needs derived from education, where Disabled children's needs were considered additional or special. Additional needs also means a teacher who was not able to support, did not understand, and a school system set up to fail Disabled young people. There is work to do within the education sector and the language imposed on young Disabled people. Access needs should not be confused with being special or additional. They are needs; everyone has needs.

Handicapable

This term was thought to be a more positive spin of the word handicap. There are different theories on the origin of the word handicap and how it became tied to Disability. First appearing in the 1900s, the word Handicap was used as a way to define physical and mental differences. Some believe it to have derived from an old saying 'hand in cap', which was a way to explain the way in which a beggar would tip their cap out to collect money. Others believe it to have stemmed from horse racing, where the fastest horses were given a handicap and would have to start further away, placing them at a disadvantage.

The origins of this word stem from disadvantage, implying that to be Disabled is to be disadvantaged. This world, although heavily considered as ableist, is still used by Disabled people worldwide who prefer this language and do view themselves as disadvantaged. If a person self-identifies this way you must respect it. It is their lived experience. The word handicapable was an attempt to make this language more positive, but it did not remove the negative connotations its predecessor carried. It had that same feeling of being disadvantaged, inadequate, a problem to be fixed. This language did not reframe the disadvantage narrative; it only deepens it and adds an extra layer of pity.

Not so fluffy euphemisms

We need to understand that when we shy away from using the words Disabled and Disability, we are allowing ableist euphemisms to downplay, eradicate, and erase the Disabled experience. This fluffy language only reinforces the historic fear and stigma that Disability or Disabled is a negative. Ableist euphemisms are not progress. They are a step backwards and they are damaging. Disability is not a negative word. Disabled is not a negative word. Do not let anyone tell you otherwise. Do not tiptoe around using one or the other. Disabled person is just as acceptable as person with Disability.

By now you are beginning to learn how ableist euphemisms grew out of stigma and fear, and that Disabled and Disability are not bad words. It is important to understand and respect both identity first and person first language.

Identity first language

'Disabled person', 'Disabled people', 'autistic person', 'Down syndrome person'. This is identity first language, which seeks to reinforce that Disability is an integral part of a person's identity. Being Disabled is not something we carry with us, but rather is a piece of our identity; it is actually society that disables us with ableism and inaccessibility. Identity first language is associated with the social model of Disability.

The social model of Disability tells us that it is society that disables us. It is the inaccessibility and lack of understanding and resources that disable an individual. Dating back to the 1970s and 1980s, the social model challenged the medical model of Disability, the prevalent model of Disability at the time. The medical model pathologised and treated Disabled people as a problem to be fixed. Fix them and you fix the problem. The social model argued against this, instead placing the responsibility on society for not having been designed for us. It saw society as seeking to oppress us and, just like sex, age, and gender oppressions, this social oppression stigmatised and marginalised Disabled people. The term Disabled person came from this model.

It is important to note that the social model of Disability was prominent in the UK and therefore today when understanding self-identity language within the UK, it's unsurprising to find the term Disabled person more commonly used than in other parts of the world. This does not mean other people in other parts of the world do not use it, but rather it is recognised in businesses in the UK and you will more likely come across Disabled person as opposed to person with Disability, which is more prominently used in the US.

Person first language

'Person with Disability', 'people with Disabilities', 'person with autism', 'person with Down syndrome'. This is person first language, which seeks to reinforce that we are people before our Disability. This language surfaced during the 20th century and was predominantly used in the US. It places the person first, and their condition/impairments second. Due to the offensive language being used at the time – such as 'retard', 'cripple', 'invalid' – advocates and scholars sought to create language that was respectful and placed the person at the centre. At this time, it was critically important to change the language used when discussing Disability, moving it from offensive, hurtful language to keep the integrity of the individual. The American with Disabilities Act 1990 further reinforced and endorsed this language, which was used in legal documents and became a widely acceptable term across the US, with many countries following suit. This filtered down into workplaces, schools, colleges, and into our everyday language.

Both identity first language and person first language have significant meaning for the person self-identifying. But it is also important to recognise and respect that there are individuals who do not opt for either person first or identity first language, and instead prefer to reclaim other terms. Language evolves, people evolve, and so does a person's choice of language when self-identifying.

Reclaiming language

There are words that an individual may use to self-identify, which may have been the cause of ableist trauma for others. These are often words that historically have been used in negative context to define Disability – words that some would consider to be outdated or offensive, but to others they give a sense of freedom and expression, a way to feel empowered by terms that have been weaponised and used against them. Reclaiming language is when an individual takes back the power of words and uses it to self-identify, bringing about a feeling of profound pride and a feeling of taking back control. Much like the word queer has been reclaimed by many within the LGBTQIA+ community, more and more individuals are using language within the Disabled community as a way to reclaim their identity.

Words like 'spastic', 'cripple', and 'retard' often dehumanised and carried negative connotations and pain for many, who had only experienced them used in situations to embarrass, insult, or injure. But some people now find solitude and strength in using these words to self-identify.

Reclaiming language is a very personal decision. It is for the individual who has the lived experience to decide which language they use to self-identify. It is their lived experience, therefore their right to identify. But what happens when one person's reclaiming language perpetrates harm for another due to its ableist historical meaning?

A person using reclaiming language is a personal choice for them, but we cannot force that choice on to groups or communities, unless the group or community agrees to use the reclaimed language in question. For example, a person with lived experience self-identifies as crippled. During a training session this person is delivering they continuously replace the words Disabled and Disability with crippled. In this instance, the individual is no longer self-identifying but rather collectively using a historically ableist term to describe a collective diverse group. This is not appropriate and will cause harm and teach non-Disabled people to think generally that it is okay to use the term.

It prepares ableism and has the potential to resurface past trauma of bullying and hurt. Self-identity is about self-identifying – no one person can speak for an entire global community and therefore it is paramount we do not use reclaiming language to describe the Disabled/Disability community.

There is no hierarchy of language when it comes to language used to self-identify. The language a person uses to self-identify is entirely their decision. It is important to respect their right to self-identity. There is no getting around it, or ignoring it. A person's choice of language is personal. Often before getting to a place of being able to self-identify, a Disabled person goes through periods of preferring or opting for one term over another.

Over time, as our feelings and view of Disability are shaped, and as we experience new things, we might opt to change or use new language. Finding the right language to self-identify with our Disability is a bit like being on a rollercoaster. There are ups and downs, and at times we think it is great, but then ahead is a big drop where suddenly we realise this was not what we signed up for.

We are on this rollercoaster for life and so it is common for people to have tried and tested different words or phrases in order to find what works for them. 'Disabled person' may have felt wrong. 'Person with Disability' may have felt icky, and so reclaiming another term might feel like the right thing. The point is we cannot prioritise one individual's self-identity and their expression over another. Questioning or invalidating a person's choice of language risks imposing harm on them. It risks affecting their self-confidence and their ability to self-identify again. You are telling them that they shouldn't use that word, or they should opt for…instead, and all it does is create doubt in this person's mind and just feeds their internalised ableism.

So never – and we mean never – challenge, question, or invalidate a person who tells you which language they use to self-identify. Respect them for sharing. If you are unclear of the language they prefer to use to self-identify, always ask, never assume.

There is power in words, and no, we aren't just talking about the power to influence or evoke emotion; we are talking about systemic power. Historically, the words in discussions about Disability were provided by non-Disabled people. This means that a lot of the language we hear or have historically experienced was led by someone without the lived experience, who did not understand what it means to be Disabled, and, more often than not, stemmed from a desire to maintain a divide, and a fear of anything that was different.

Sugar-coated euphemisms like differently abled or different abilities have become safer, preferable terms to use, when in reality if you ask the majority of Disabled people, they will tell you that this language is ableist. This language seeks to treat Disabled people as different, as special, as a source of pity or inspiration. This is why it is essential to listen to those with lived experiences, and ask their preferred way to self-identify; to give the power back to Disabled people to make choices about their lives. It is important to respect the language they use, and remember that non-Disabled people should not be holding conversations about language without the presence of Disabled voices to guiding them. While we need allies, we also need to ensure that the allies know to pass the mic.

Comparative language

You might have noticed that throughout this book we use the terms 'non-Disabled person' or 'people without Disabilities'. We do this in order to help change the narrative that being Disabled makes us abnormal, because that's what we hear in society: 'they are normal', meaning they don't have a Disability, and 'they are special', meaning they are Disabled. Society uses divisive language stemming from its history of excluding Disabled people. And so, when making a comparison between Disabled people and people without Disabilities, please do so without creating a harmful comparison.

Able-bodied

This term implies that every Disabled person does not have an able body. By now, you know that Disability is diverse and there is no one appearance and no one experience. When non-Disabled people are described as able-bodied, this shows a failure to understand and respect the diversity of Disability. 'Able-bodied' creates a binary difference between what is able and what is not able. It paints an unequitable comparison between Disabled people and our non-Disabled peers. This term does not accurately define the difference between a Disabled person or a non-Disabled person. The power dynamics at play when using this term shape the thinking of what a normal body should be, disregarding the many diverse differences between all bodies, not just Disabled bodies.

Normal

What even is normal? Can anyone actually define what it means? Your version of normal is different from everyone else's around you. When you refer to non-Disabled people as normal, you are creating a distinction that Disability is therefore abnormal. Less desirable, less attractive, less than ideal. You impose the belief that Disability is indifferent, when in reality there are more than 1.7 billion Disabled people globally – more than a quarter of the world population – so how can being Disabled make us abnormal when it is clearly part of the human experience? The word normal creates a benchmark for a standard that is unachievable, resulting in Disabled people being viewed as less than or a deviant of what normal should be. What is considered normal in one culture is not in another, and what is normal to one person may not be to another. It is vital to move away from referring to non-Disabled people as normal because it does not exist. It is a false standard. And it is belittling.

When using language that seeks to compare Disabled people to non-Disabled people rather than using words that divide or seek to reinforce differences, simply say non-Disabled person or person without Disabilities. This does not create an inequitable comparison, it is not demonising Disability, and it is not creating a hierarchy or a false standard.

Dismissive language

On the flip side of this we also have to address outright ignorance. When a non-Disabled person makes comments such as, 'Everyone is a little Disabled/autistic/ADHD...', this ableism is ignorance. It completely disregards a Disabled person's lived experiences and dismisses the very real challenges they have had to overcome or endure. Everyone is not a little bit Disabled. Not every person faces inaccessible barriers daily. Not every person has to enter a space fearful of requesting their access needs or the need to self-identify. The privilege in statements such as these is staggering. To centre yourself in another's oppression is privilege at its strongest. It is no better than those who attempt to downplay racism with ignorant comments such as, 'I don't see colour.' This type of ignorance takes so much energy to respond to. It is just a privileged individual declaring themselves the most amazing inclusive ally, but yet trying to centre themselves in the identify of those they claim to show allyship for. Do not fall into this trap. Yes, not every Disability is visible, not every Disability is apparent, but that does not mean you do not see Disability.

Ableism has become so ingrained in everyday language that some people, when told that what they have said was ableist, refuse to believe it and so they push back, opting instead to become defensive, aggressive, or argumentative: 'Stop being so woke', 'You are being so sensitive', 'I have Disabled friends, I cannot be ableist.' These sorts of comments are part of the everyday challenges in calling out ableist language. People do this because they do not understand, and they fear that which they do not understand. They believe themselves to be right, and it is easy to feel right in a society that provides so much conflicting information. Children use ableist language, adults use ableist language, Disabled people use ableist language. We all have unlearning to do.

  " Language is powerful. It has the power to shape thoughts and affect actions. It has the power to shift perspectives.

Think of it like a tool that can build or break or even like social media that can connect and empower or divide and dehumanise. It is something that many of us take for granted but it is immensely powerful, which is precisely why we should practise caution while drafting our language, as sometimes the words we use as part of our language can stem from ableism.

Ableism has been indoctrinated generationally into most if not all of us through our systems, our environments, and our societies, so much so that sometimes we exercise ableism unconsciously without even knowing that what we are saying or doing is ableist. In fact, many of us have internalised ableism without even realising it.

An example of ableist language which has become a norm and is usually meant as a 'compliment' is, 'Don't worry, you don't look autistic' or another example when it comes to sensory needs is, 'It is not that loud, come on!'

Such responses foster internalised ableism, not just in you but also in others.

Internalised ableism can sometimes look like believing that you have to complete a task or do something to be of value.

Hence, if the language you are using is ableist, it's going to increase internalised ableism in many neurodivergent and otherwise Disabled people. You have to change your language to break the cycle of generational ableism. Change your words. Change your language. Be a change maker by being anti-ableist. 99

– Samar Waqar, Founder and Executive Director of Kind Theory, and a neurodiversity and DEI-AB (diversity, equity, inclusion, accessibility, and belonging) expert

Ableism is evident not just in how we talk about Disability or how people self-identify. It is also in the responses Disabled people have to endure when they share their lived experiences: language that seeks to make only the non-Disabled person more comfortable; language that denounces, overlooks, dismisses, or eradicates Disability. Let's look at some of the ableist responses we receive on sharing our Disabilities.

Imagine that a Disabled person has opened up and self-identified. They found the courage and confidence to share but unfortunately for them, the vast majority of responses to this sharing consist of well-meaning intent, wrapped up in an ableist bow, perpetrating harm in the words used.

I don't see you as Disabled

Disability is not always visible. You do not need to try to assure us you see us as a person. We can be a person and be Disabled at the same time. When you tell us you don't see us as Disabled, you're telling us you don't believe us. You are telling us that our experiences do not matter. The challenges we face do not matter. This response is ignorant of what it means to be Disabled and the diversity of Disability.

But you look so healthy

Disability is not an illness, or at least not all illnesses are a Disability. While Disabled people may have chronic conditions, sickness, and so on, being unhealthy is not a qualifier for Disability. When you assume that Disability only equates to illness you overlook the diverse differences of Disability. We know by now that Disability does not have one appearance. A Disabled person may feel bursting with energy one day, only for fatigue, burnout, or their conditions/impairments to flare up on another day. Disability is not restricted to appearance. It is important to move away from language that reinforces Disability as an easily recognisable thing. It is better to assume someone is Disabled, rather than creating false criteria to identify those that are. You don't look healthy, but does that make you Disabled? No, it does not, but do you understand now how silly that sounds?

You can't be Disabled!

Why can't we be? Responding in shock, horror, or gasps that we can't be is honestly just the most belittling experience. Who sets the criteria of how a person can and cannot be Disabled? What makes you the expert who can tell a person they can or cannot be Disabled? This ableist response stems from, you guessed it, the belief that Disability is only visible, that if you don't look the part, you can't be. If you don't fit this person's bias view, then you, my friend, can't be Disabled. When someone shares their sexuality or gender, do you exclaim,

'Oh you can't be?' No, you don't, or at least you should not. Why is it acceptable to remove a piece of a person's identity after they have just shared something sensitive? Let's stop the, 'You can't be' and start with the, 'Thank you for sharing.'

You don't look Disabled

Much like telling a person they can't be Disabled, 'you don't look it' completely misses the mark on recognising and understanding the diversity of Disability. It will always be an inaccurate way to measure if a person is Disabled or not because we know Disability is not always visible. When you respond with 'You don't look it', we might have to start replying with, 'And you don't look ableist but yet here we are in this uncomfortable situation.'

You are so inspirational

On sharing our Disability and being confronted with, 'You're so inspirational', it's hard not to feel patronised. This is a stranger who does not know us, does not know our achievements, does not know anything about us other than this piece of our identity we have shared, most likely because we had no choice at the time. This is a person proclaiming how inspirational we are just because we happen to be Disabled. This response is so cringy that even writing about it makes us feel nauseous. A person is not inspirational simply for being born or acquiring Disability. It is a piece of our identity, one of many pieces. Does having green eyes make a person inspirational? No, it does not, and it's ludicrous to suggest it would. But yet when we share our Disability, people patronise us by calling us inspirational.

This language stems from Disability inspiration porn and has been adopted into mainstream media. If you pick up a paper and find a story about a Disabled person, note how the language used is all about how inspirational this person is. The language is not empowering but rather seeks to use the Disabled person as inspiration porn. 'Well, if they can do it, you can.' Judge a person by their actions, accomplishments, and achievements. Yes, a person may inspire you because of the things they have done or said, but do not let it be because they shared their Disabilities. Do not let this be your response – all it does is inspire us to shy away from sharing again.

I am so sorry

Why are you sorry? You do not need to apologise for our lived experience. Unless you have offended, insulted, used outdated language, used euphemisms, or you have used language to cause offence intentionally, you do not need to be sorry when we share. It is pity wrapped up in ableist clothing. We do not need your pity. We do not need you to suddenly change your tone of voice as you hand out your condolences. Pity is not empathy. Your pity is condescending, demeaning, uncomfortable. It tells us that to be Disabled is not a good thing, but a bad, negative thing. We discussed earlier how privilege can intervene in your response. When you apologise after we have shared, you are only making yourself comfortable and centring yourself in our self-identity.

When responding to a person self-identifying, strive for positive engagement. Try to make it a response that encourages the person to continue the conversation. Thank the person for self-identifying; ask them if there is a more accessible way to communicate or if they have any access needs. Do not seek to question, invalidate, or belittle their experience. Show respect, as you would towards the language the person uses to self-identify.

Choosing better words and phrases

We have to be able to shake off the stigma and fear of talking about Disability and we need to move away from language that is outdated, offensive, overlooks, or dismisses Disability. This language has become so intertwined in everyday speech. Words like 'lame', 'crazy', 'retard', 'spaz', 'midget', 'dumb' are bandied about, disregarding the historic context and stigmatisation, just used as throwaway comments and insults. People aren't aware and so they continue to use them, making jokes with friends, or insulting anyone who is different from or less than their own version of what normal is. And while of course, we discussed the need to respect an individual who self-identifies with reclaiming language, it does not make it okay for non-Disabled people and Disabled people to use these terms in their everyday language.

There is a difference between a Disabled person reclaiming the word 'spaz', and a non-Disabled person calling his friend a spaz in anger. One is an individual self-identifying with a word which empowers them; the other is offensive and meant to degrade. Let's look at everyday ableism and the terms we can use instead.

Terms/words to avoid	Instead, say
'Special' 'Differently abled' 'Handicap' 'Retard' 'Spaz' 'Handicapable' Challenged' 'Special'	'Disabled person' 'Person with Disability' 'How do you prefer to self-identify?'
'Normal' 'Healthy' 'Able-bodied'	'Non-Disabled person' 'Person without Disability'
'Special needs' 'Additional needs'	'Access needs' 'Accessibility needs' 'Adjustment/Accommodation needs' 'Needs'
'Wheelchair bound' 'Confined to a wheelchair'	'Wheelchair user' 'Person using a wheelchair' 'Uses a wheelchair'
'Midget' 'Dwarf'	'Person with dwarfism' 'Little person'

'Crippled' 'Lame' 'Deformed' 'Spastic'	'Has a physical Disability' 'Disabled person' 'Person with Disability' *(Unless used as self-identification language)*
'Disabled bathroom' 'Disability bathroom'	'Accessible bathroom' 'Bathroom for access needs'
'Crazy' 'Insane' *(When used as an adjective)*	'Unreal' 'Frustrating' 'Unbelievable' 'Wild' 'Unexpected'
'Dumb'	'Uninformed' 'Misguided' 'Silly'
'Suffers with' 'Affected by' 'Victim of'	'Is Disabled' 'Has a Disability'
'High functioning' 'Low functioning'	'Person who is able to' 'Person who is unable to'
'Psycho'	'Unstable' 'Erratic'
'Tone Deaf'	'Insensitive' 'Uncaring' 'Inconsiderate'
'Crazy'	'Overwhelmed'
'Blind spot'	'Out of my vision' 'Did not see it'
'Slow' 'Simple' 'Stupid'	'Unaware' 'Do not understand'
'Fell on Deaf ears'	'I did not hear you' 'I don't understand'
'They're so bipolar' *(When used to describe a person)*	'They're moody' 'They are up and down'
'They're so OCD' *(Obsessive compulsive disorder. When used to describe a person)*	'They are very neat' 'They are well organised'

This list is not exhaustive.

Unlearning ableism is more than challenging or changing our own language; it is about being open to understanding people are going to say the wrong thing. People are going to make mistakes because they are not provided with the knowledge or resources to know better.

It is important to create safe spaces for people to be able to call out ableism, and for people to learn that what they have said is inappropriate. Everyone needs to be open to unlearning and learning. If a person says or does the wrong thing, if they do so accidentally or indirectly cause offence, they must be given the opportunity to learn from it. Be patient; show understanding, and be open to helping others unlearn. Stop talking about Disability as though it is a big bad thing. Change your tone of voice from pity to reassurance, from fear to acceptance.

Yes, being Disabled means a person might experience challenges; yes, they have to deal with ableism; and of course, yes, they will have days where it is frustrating and exhausting and they want to scream into their pillow. Disabled people are people. They do not want to be ostracised by your choice of language, or your preferred method of communication.

We think of language and we think of voice, we think of speaking, we do not think of d/Deaf people, who sign, or other Disabled people who use voice assistant technologies and so on. It is important to understand that language is communication, and communication needs to respect and include Disabled people with diverse ways of communicating.

> 66 Fewer than 5% of d/Deaf and hard of hearing people in the US use sign language. People seem to think most of us are fluent in it. We're not. It's very uncommon.

Say these words without sound: mom, pop, mop, bop, bob, mob. They all look the same on the lips. My bionic ear detects the difference between puh, muh, and buh. Same with -op and -ob.

When you meet a d/Deaf person or someone who doesn't understand you, offer to communicate in other ways. Try to move away from defaulting to only one method of communication: voicing.

I love meeting people and having conversations. But I feel as if people don't want to approach me and they have walls up. If you're concerned that I won't understand you or you want to be proactive, offer to rephrase things, write them down, or use a smartphone.

State this upfront. Then, it'll be easier for me to ask. It's hard to ask people to repeat more than once. If that doesn't work, social bluffing comes in and I start smiling and nodding.

On a captioned video call, someone said they had an accent and to please let them know if I needed anything repeated or typed into the chatbox. I said the same goes for them too. Do the same for others, regardless of speech patterns or accent.

Another time, someone asked if I wanted an interpreter. They asked if I had a preferred interpreter and that they had an interpreting agency they used.

I love this for three reasons:

1. They asked instead of assuming I used sign language.

2. They gave me the opportunity to choose their preferred interpreter.

3. They mentioned they had one so I didn't feel responsible for naming an interpreter if they didn't have one in mind. **99**

– Meryl K. Evans, speaker and consultant, https://meryl.net

Disabled people want to be included in the conversation. We want to be able to share our views openly and accessibly, without fear! We do not want to have to squirm inside as you say something offensive, degrading, or belittling. We want to feel included. We want to engage in a conversation where we don't have to suddenly stop because yet again ableism has popped up in conversation.

That was a lot to digest and a lot to get your head around, but we hope by now you are learning that ableism, even in language, has the means to oppress and harm Disabled people. Even when people are not seeking to cause harm, ableism is there ingrained in thoughts, hidden in words, and stuck in learned behaviours.

66 'Language is the road map of a culture. It tells you where its people come from and where they are going' (Rita Mae Brown). The language we use not only describes the world, it shapes it. Words like 'Disabled' and 'Disability' are often avoided or replaced with euphemisms such as 'differently abled'. This avoidance implies that Disability is something shameful, less than, and perpetuates harmful stereotypes. Language shapes the zeitgeist, moulding societal norms and attitudes. By reclaiming the word Disabled, we push back against aged, outdated, and frankly harmful narratives which are rooted in pity and fear. But here's the truth: reclaiming Disabled isn't just important, it is revolutionary. Reclamation of Disabled/Disability disrupts these cycles which are steeped in unease. When you say 'I'm

Disabled' loud and proud, you reject the idea that being Disabled is inherently bad. You challenge the stigma that tries to paint Disability as a deficit or something to 'overcome'. Instead, you declare it as a part of who you are, and that's empowering. It says, 'This is my identity, and there is nothing wrong with it.' By owning the term Disabled we shift the narrative from pity to pride. Words have power and when we use them intentionally, we create a culture that uplifts and values Disabled people. It's not something we should hide or whisper – it's a part of the human experience. 99

– Brooke Millhouse, Founder, Disabled & Proud Podcast

Unlearning ableism from our language will take time. It takes a heck of a lot of patience, but it also starts with individuals being able to safely call it out. So, if you do anything after this chapter, tell someone what you've learned. Do a post on your social media. Tell your friends or family. Help destigmatise Disability. Adopt inclusive language and, most of all, be open to challenging the ableist language in our workplaces, education, healthcare, and across all corners of our society.

CHAPTER 8

Unlearning Ableism: Legislation, Rights, and Policy

> There exists a global network of laws, policies, and legislations that exist on domestic and international levels, which are theoretically designed to protect Disabled people in equity of access to opportunity, participation, and protection. However, a global failure of enforcement, loopholes, and lack of prioritisation means that Disabled people are not receiving the benefits of these protections. Politicians are still making decisions without correct consultation, Disabled people are shockingly underrepresented among our law-makers, oh and some Disabled people can't even vote due to inaccessibility. Nothing about us without us? Disabled rights are fundamental human rights – not privileges or favours – so why oh why are we still fighting for our basic rights to be fulfilled?

An introduction to policy, legislation, and Disability rights

Policy, legislation, and Disability rights are the scary and intimidating important stuff, right? It is perfectly natural to feel slightly nervous when we start talking about these kinds of things, as, let's be honest, it can often feel very overwhelming. What laws are we bound by? How are we protected? What laws govern how other people must behave? It's a whole wide blue, and very choppy, sea of conversation that is widely neglected. It is perfectly normal to not know the answers to these questions. When you become Disabled or start learning about Disability, the United Nations Convention on the Rights of Persons with Disabilities is not automatically downloaded to our brains and we all become legal whizzes, but it is crucial that we learn the answers to these questions in our own personal journeys to unlearn ableism.

(A small disclaimer: We can't possibly cover every country's Disability policy, legislation, and rights in one chapter – we would need a whole series of encyclopedias to cover it all – so we are going to take one country, the UK, to use as an example that provides a reflective case study of what is really going on.)

So why is it so important to become legal eagles? It's a simple answer really. It will help to ensure that:

- Disabled people feel empowered to call out behaviour that is discriminatory

- judicial systems set precedence for those who challenge the status quo

- Disabled people are able to protect themselves and their safety

- Disabled people know their rights and what they can ask for

- non-Disabled people, organisations, and charities behave in the way set out in law.

In developing a collective understanding of the rules that tell us all what to do and what not to do, legislations and policies are massive components in breaking down systemic ableism. A really good example to give here is the right to reasonable adjustments in the workplace (which we will get into later into this chapter), knowing what we can ask for, why we can ask for it, and that it has to be given.

> 66 When developing policy and legislation for the Government of Gibraltar, I always begin with Marshall Ganz's Public Narrative theory whereby three key factors need to be taken into consideration:
>
> 1. The story of self: How does this issue affect my son (he has a Disability) and my family? What would we like to see happen?
>
> 2. The story of us: How is this issue affecting others in the community? What are the shared goals within the community?
>
> 3. The story of now: What action is necessary? What must be included in the new policy or legislation?
>
> Following this methodology ensures that there is direct consultation with persons with lived experience and that policy is developed from what the people truly need. In the early days, I was worried about critique and I would dwell on how to make it perfect prior to implementation; however, the most important lesson I have learned along the way is that policy and legislation will never be perfect! Disability is wide-ranging and one size does not fit all, so constant review is necessary. It is also imperative to implement measures of control directly into the policy or legislation; for example, having tests of reasonability for issues surrounding reasonable adjustments, and implementing checks and balances. I have come to realise that not publishing

or implementing a policy because I didn't think it was perfect is perhaps more damaging than not getting it right. In Gibraltar and across the rest of the world, we are striving for a culture change away from ableism. Policies are necessary to create this culture change and formalise practices, because it is a human right and not just because it is the right thing to do. People come and go; however, policies remain. 〞

– **Jenny Victory, Head of Disability Office, Government of Gibraltar**

What is legally counted as ableism?

What does this all mean in practice? We're about to learn what is legally counted as ableism, so that we know our rights when violated and learn about our legal responsibilities to others. By knowing our rights and laws we can tackle ableism head on. And quite blatantly the question here arises as to why we aren't already being taught all of this in schools, our workplaces, or even by the people around us? (But that's a topic for another chapter, which we will dive into soon.)

Unfortunately, as it stands, the laws that are designed to protect Disabled people are being violated left, right, and center, because not only do Disabled people not know their rights, but rather worryingly, organisations and individuals don't know what they are supposed to be doing, by law!

And this isn't necessarily our fault; we aren't teaching Disabled children or adults their rights in schools or workplaces, we aren't embedding Disability laws into human resources practices, and nine times out of ten we have to ask, as we are never offered. However, we all have an individual and collective responsibility to take accountability of our actions and biases, and with conscious positive intent start to learn and develop our understanding. But panic not, through this chapter we are going to undo all of this, strip it back to basics, and get ourselves back on track.

It is, however, very important to acknowledge here that the laws and policies that we have at the moment are not perfect. There is still so much to do to make sure our legislation is properly working to protect people. There are still loopholes and gaps that need closing. This does not in any way mean that knowing our rights and protections, or knowing how to treat Disabled people by law, is invalidated – actually quite the opposite – what it means is that together as a united force we can call out these gaps in protection and work together to build better rights for the future.

In Chapter 1, we learned about the social model of Disability and the medical model of Disability and why it is so important that we follow the social model. We need to make sure that rather than our laws not being ableist, they are anti-ableist, proactive not reactive, and actively seek movement forward to embed the principles of unlearning ableism (but we might be a little biased towards that).

So with all that, let us begin

What are we actually talking about when we talk about legislation, policy, and Disability rights? What do these words actually mean?

Legislation, according to the Cambridge Dictionary, 'is a law or set of laws suggested by a Government and made official by a Parliament' (Cambridge Dictionary, n.d.b).*

*Disclaimer: In countries without democratic leadership or established Parliaments, laws can be passed with executive decision based on the decision of a single person or a small group of individuals.

And what is a law? A law is a set standard of behaviour, a procedure or action stating what is correct and incorrect. Legislation can come from Parliament at home or from international bodies such as the United Nations, which designs conventions that countries then take and put them into their own legal systems. These networks of laws are then used by the judiciary (the courts and legal system) to make decisions about the cases brought forward.

Policy is points of action – the manual of how we behave, adopted by organisations, individuals, and governing bodies; for example, welfare schemes, language developments, practices and behaviours, strategies and legislation. Policy is 'a set of ideas or a plan of what to do in particular situations that has been agreed to officially by a group of people, a business organisation, a government, or a political party', as defined by Cambridge Dictionary (n.d.).

Disability rights are references to the collective of laws and policies which protect Disabled people from discrimination and ableism.

So all of these three things – legislation, policy, Disability rights – are designed to ensure equal opportunity, participation, access, and fair treatment for Disabled people.

Let's start off with some definitions so we can get our heads around everything we are about to discuss.

What is the legal definition of Disability, ableism, and discrimination?

A Disability is when you have 'a physical or mental impairment' that has a 'substantial' and 'long-term' negative effect on your ability to carry out normal daily activities. Substantial means it is more than 'minor', so your condition really affects how you would complete daily tasks compared to non-Disabled people. And long-term means it is older than 12 months or a health condition that develops as a result of another condition. This definition also includes 'progressive conditions' – things that get worse over time – and you automatically receive Disability rights from the day of your diagnosis (this is all found in the Equality Act, which we are about to explore).

There are also lots of pieces of international law which define Disability. For example, the United Nations (2006) says 'persons with Disabilities include those who have long-term physical, mental, intellectual or sensory impairments which in interaction with various barriers may hinder their full and effective participation in society on an equal basis with others'.

The definition of ableism is 'the less favourable treatment of Disabled people in favour of those who do not have a Disability' (Oxford English Dictionary, n.d.a).

And the definition of discrimination is 'the unjust or prejudicial treatment of different categories of people, especially on the grounds of ethnicity, age, sex, or Disability' (Oxford English Dictionary, n.d.c).

So, when we say ableism (which we have quite a bit, so we definitely need to learn this one early!), we are referring to the specific type of discrimination that Disabled people face.

The Equality Act of 2010

Off we go, let's kick it off and start with a big one – the Equality Act of 2010, which replaced and zhuzhed up the Disability Discrimination Act of 1995 and 2005. The Equality Act is the biggest and most important piece of legislation we have which secures accessibility, equality, and the prevention of discrimination against Disabled people in law.

The Equality Act intends to prevent people being denied or receiving a lesser service as a direct result of their Disability. The Act also encompasses 'associates' of Disabled people, such as carers, parents, and guardians.

The Equality Act explicitly says that under no circumstance is a Disabled person to be placed at a disadvantage, treated unfavourably, or discriminated against due to actions relating to their Disability; this can be trifold in its existence, so here we are talking about direct discrimination, indirect discrimination, or failure to make reasonable adjustments.

What do we mean by direct and indirect discrimination – isn't discrimination just one thing? Not at all. Like all types of discrimination, not just Disability related, it can take various different formats.

Direct discrimination is when a person is treated unfavourably by another person because of their Disability; for example, if someone isn't hired for a job just because they are a Disabled person.

Indirect discrimination is when a Disabled person is treated unfavourably by another due to certain circumstances that have a negative impact on them. This one is a little trickier to recognise sometimes, but going back to our previous example of recruitment, an indirect discrimination is where the job application isn't accessible or accessible formats of the job description haven't been made available.

Both indirect and direct discrimination are illegal. Most people only think of direct discrimination as being a big no-no but it goes much further than you think. There is an exception here, which is worth noting. Indirect and direct discrimination are permitted if the proportionate objective demonstration can be shown. For example, the armed forces have very strict health requirements to be able to join in order to protect life and safety. While exceptions like these are typically very few and far between, it is important to note that it can sometimes happen.

The Equality Act is legally binding; this means that you have to adhere to it, always. So, how does this relate to ableism?

Well quite clearly if we don't want to break the law, we all need to be thinking about how our actions might directly or indirectly discriminate against someone.

Defining direct and indirect forms of discrimination

Macroaggressions: Large systematic oppressions of Disabled people which reinforce discrimination that favours non-Disabled people. Examples include: policies that don't include Disabled people, segregation, or preventing Disabled people from participating in certain activities.

Microaggressions: Things that make a Disabled person feel uncomfortable or marginalised. Examples include: how we speak about and to Disabled people, how we treat people, misconceptions, and stereotypes.

Understanding these forms of aggressions, both of which are illegal under the Equality Act we should add, helps us identify our own behaviours and our behaviours as a society.

Conscious bias: Sometimes also known as an 'explicit' bias, where you are conscious with the decisions and actions you are making, in other words you know you're doing it, acting with intention.

An example of this might be not being friends with someone because they are Disabled, or shouting at a Disabled person in the street.

Unconscious bias: Similar to what we have already discussed, where a person holds biases towards Disabled people without even realising they are doing it. For example: not having an accessible website, planning an event without thinking about accessibility, contributing to Disability inspiration porn, or speaking to Disabled people as if they are children (infantilisation, which happens all the time). Unconscious bias is triggered because we automatically make quick judgements based on our experiences and what we know. It is a massive contributor to ableist inequalities, and this is why education and awareness is so important.

Under the Equality Act, Disabled people are also able to report acts of discrimination as hate crime to the police. Sometimes, even though we think we aren't ableist because we don't actively hate Disabled people or would never intentionally do anything to discriminate against someone, our unconscious actions are ableist. We mentioned some of these in our introduction, but the language we use, how we address accessibility, intersectionality, and all of the chapters we discuss across all different areas in this book, play a part in this conversation (and a key component in our journey to unlearning ableism).

Positive action and reasonable adjustments

The Equality Act also teaches us two other really important anti-ableist points. First, the necessity of something called positive action, a similar phrase to one you will see us using time and time again throughout this book; being proactive and not reactive.

Positive action means that Disabled people should not have to be constantly asking for things, requesting reasonable adjustments (examples of this include a British Sign Language interpreter, accessible and adaptive technology, or specialist equipment), or appealing for accessibility to be put in place. This is also known as pre-emptive duty – we must always be expecting Disabled participation and act accordingly. Another turn of phrase you will see us use a lot is 'from the point of design'. This means that by law we are digging down in an attempt to remove ableism which is buried deep within our society, always fostering an environment which encourages and does not prevent Disabled participation.

And our second one? Reasonable adjustments, another big topic we need to address in our unlearning of ableism. Reasonable adjustment means that you legally must ensure that Disabled people can access employment, services, activities, education (the full works), and if they are not able to, adjustments have to be made or additional provisions supplied to prevent a 'substantial disadvantage'. This isn't just applicable to the workplace, but to education as well.

For the schooling of Disabled children, this means that 'all publicly funded preschools, nurseries, state schools, and local authorities must try to identify and help assess children with special educational needs and disabilities (SEND)' and 'all universities and higher education colleges should have a person in charge of Disability issues that you can talk to about the support they offer' (UK Government, 2010).

Removing ableist barriers

Disabled people have equal rights to non-Disabled people (the equality of opportunity rhetoric, which we will be covering in Chapter 10 on representation), to be able to use, access, participate, and enjoy the same services through the removal of barriers.

Well actually this is brilliant news for our collective effort to banish ableism. What the law is saying is if you make something new you must put the barriers down for Disabled people, but if something already exists and has barriers for Disabled people, it is your duty to get rid of them. What does this mean on the other side of the conversation for Disabled people? It means that we are protected. By understanding this part of the law we know we can make requests for adjustments, hold people to account, call out discrimination, and legally take action. We love a bit of accountability! The Equality Act is a 'binding' act which means, well simply, do it or face the consequences.

Access to Work scheme

The Access to Work scheme also ties in nicely here as yet another issue regarding the rights for Disabled people to ensure that barriers can be broken down, specifically in employment. Access to Work is a grant, communications, and advice scheme run by the Government for Disabled people offering three types of services; 'a grant to help pay for practical support with your work, advice about managing your mental health at work, and money to pay for communication support at job interviews' (UK Government, n.d.). Examples of the Access to Work scheme in practice might be:

- hiring a virtual assistant
- grants for interpreters
- transport adaptations
- providing accessible technology.

This is not means-tested (meaning it doesn't matter how much you earn, you are still eligible) and does not affect any of the other benefits that you might receive. Access to Work is not only valuable for Disabled people to know our rights and what we can ask for, but also for non-Disabled people struggling to break down barriers they might have within their companies to encourage better internal Disabled representation. And the UK isn't the only one to have a scheme like this; America has the Equal Employment Opportunity Commission.

Anticipatory duty

Something we should also mention here is our wonderful friend 'anticipatory duty', which, as well as being written into legislation, also provides enormous guidance on how we should all be acting towards our journeys in unlearning ableism.

Anticipatory duty is where organisations must act in a way which expects Disability and adjustments, making them in advance if they know that there are barriers that are going to put people at a substantial disadvantage compared to non-Disabled people. Employers have a responsibility to make sure that Disabled people can access jobs, education, and services as easily as non-Disabled people. This is known as the 'duty to make reasonable adjustments'. Disabled people can experience discrimination if the employer or organisation doesn't make a reasonable adjustment. This is known as a 'failure to make reasonable adjustments'.

Public Sector Equality Duty

In 2011, the UK Government went even further with the Equality Act and created something called the Public Sector Equality Duty (PSED). This says that any public authorities – things like venues, museums, local governments, and national programmes – have a duty to act in a way that enhances opportunity and participation of all people to prevent discrimination (and for the purposes of this book, ableism).

This was excellent news, and provides even more opportunity to hold people to account and to enforce our Disabled rights. Again, just like the Equality Act, the PSED is compulsory, so our public bodies (which is a body which is publicly funded or run by a government service) must make sure their actions, policies, and managerial decisions are actively working to break down ableism and barriers of participation for Disabled people. This is done through three set actions of:

- removing or minimising disadvantages suffered by people due to their characteristics

- meeting the needs of people from protected groups where these are different from the needs of other people

- encouraging people from protected groups to participate in public life or other activities where their participation is disproportionately low.

Active anti-ableism!

The Human Rights Act of 1998

Moving on to another really key piece of law, we should all be familiar with the Human Rights Act of 1998 (UK Government, 1998). This incorporates the European Convention on Human Rights into our laws (Council of Europe, 1950), which means we took the writings of the European law and copied them into ours, creating that double layer of protection. We can hear you all asking, but what about Brexit; surely we don't have this any more? This Convention is totally separate from the European Union and is very much still around and designed to protect human rights and political freedoms right across Europe; it's definitely not a European Union thing.

The Human Rights Act and the European Convention on Human Rights have many sections about the protection of equality for all people, which are applicable to Disabled people.

This means that not only can you take someone to court here, but you can also up-the-ante and take someone to the European Courts of Justice (Europe's high court, effectively with the ultimate say) when something really awful has happened. Again, despite Brexit, this does not prevent UK eligibility to submit a case to the European Court of Human Rights, due to the legal separation of these two entities.

As we said, these two legislative pieces are huge, so let's just explore one example to begin with so we don't massively overwhelm ourselves with too much information across thousands and thousands of pages.

In the Human Rights Act, Article 14 describes 'protection from discrimination' both direct and indirect. This means that all of the Articles (which really just means sections) of this piece of law are applicable to Disability, just as much as they are applicable to other elements of a person's identity, such as their gender, religion, and race. Once again, those who fail to adhere to this principle for the prevention and eradication of ableism are legally liable. Both the European Convention on Human Rights and the Human Rights Act provide legislative protection for the enforcement of accessibility and the promotion of Disabled inclusion.

What we are aiming to show, by learning about our legislation, policy, and Disability rights, is that Disabled people are protected and able to hold others to account if they behave in a discriminatory way. There is no such thing as a small discrimination – all discrimination is illegal, so heads up non-Disabled people and organisations, this is a reminder to you of what you must legally be doing.

The United Nations

It's not just Europe that has banded together to create laws which protect Disabled people and call for equality and the removal of ableism; the world collectively is doing it too – incoming, the United Nations. The United Nations is a diplomatic and political international organisation whose stated purposes are to 'maintain international peace and security', 'develop friendly relations among nations', achieve 'international cooperation', and serve as a centre for 'harmonising the actions of nations' (United Nations, 1945). Think of the UN as the world (well some of it) coming together to standardise human rights, and, among other things, creating guidance on what is right and what is wrong, which countries can then take away and adopt into their own principles, as well as following the laws they set.

We also need to know about the United Nations Convention on the Rights of Persons with Disabilities (UNCRPD) which the UK ratified (a fancy word for adopted) in 2009. The purpose of this Convention is: 'to promote, protect and ensure the full and equal enjoyment of all human rights and fundamental freedoms by all persons with disabilities, and to promote respect for their inherent dignity' (United Nations, 2006). This Convention has 50 different Articles which cover all aspects of life from justice, to children, to privacy, education, and health.

In the Convention, it says:

> People are free to make their own choices, no one will be discriminated against, Disabled people have the same rights to be included in society as anybody else, Disabled people are to be respected for who they are, everyone should have equal opportunities, everyone should have equal access, and Disabled children should be respected for who they are as they grow up. (United Nations, 2006)

It also states that countries should make sure that Disabled people actually do get treated equally by making rules and laws to give Disabled people their rights and changing any laws that aren't fair, making sure the rights of Disabled people to be treated equally are included in all policies, doing as much as they can to make sure no one discriminates against Disabled people, making sure things are designed for everyone to use or can be easily changed, using new technology to help Disabled people, giving accessible information to Disabled people about the things that will help them, and training relevant people about this agreement.

Once again, similar to other international law we have learned about already, the UNCRPD is legally binding and sets forward the 'minimum standards for rights of people with disabilities', for the improvement of accessibility, discrimination, and equality of participation opportunity. The UNCRPD is important to know about because not only do we have laws that bind individuals, organisations, and bodies, we also have legislation about how we are tackling ableism as a country! On the world stage, each of its signatory countries are held accountable. As Disabled people, we also have the right to hold our country to account for its actions.

When we are talking about Disability rights, this is the big one – the beefy point of back-referral, the grail if you will: the UNCRPD aims to change attitudes and approaches to persons with Disabilities, moving countries from the medical to social model of Disability.

It stops people from viewing persons with Disabilities as 'objects' of charity, medical treatment, and social protection and towards viewing them as 'subjects' with rights, who are capable of claiming those rights and making decisions for their lives based on their free and informed consent, and being active members of society.

The UNCRPD still holds the title of the highest number of signatories in history to a UN Convention on its opening day, and the fastest negotiated human rights treaty. Gibraltar is currently on a journey to become a signatory on the UNCRPD, and therefore implementing its Articles through legislative change and The National Disability strategy.

The Convention is the first international human rights treaty which explicitly identifies the rights of persons with Disabilities as well as the obligations on Parliaments to promote, protect, and ensure those rights. It reaffirms that all persons with all types of Disabilities must enjoy the same human rights, opportunities, participations, and fundamental freedoms as non-Disabled people.

In its 'Articles', the Convention clarifies the rights of persons with Disabilities and identifies areas where adaptations have to be made for persons with Disabilities to effectively exercise their rights, and areas where their rights have been violated, and where protection of rights must be reinforced.

All members of society should have the same human rights; they include civil, cultural, economic, political, and social rights. Examples include equality before the law without discrimination; right to life; liberty, and security of the person; equal recognition before the law and legal capacity; right to live in the community; freedom of expression and opinion; right to education, health, work, and an adequate standard of living; right to participate in political and public life; and right to participate in cultural life.

All individuals with Disabilities have the right to be free from discrimination in the enjoyment of their rights. This includes the right to be free from discrimination on the basis of any other intersectional basis such as race, colour, sex, language, religion, political or other opinion, national, or social origin, property, birth, or other status.

The Convention identifies three different categories of obligations: general obligations, enabling measures and specific obligations on states in relation to the rights of persons with Disabilities.

General obligations mean that states (countries) have to:

- adopt legislation and administrative measures to promote the human rights of persons with Disabilities

- adopt legislative and other measures to abolish discrimination

- protect and promote the rights of persons with Disabilities in all policies and programmes

- stop any practice that breaches the rights of persons with Disabilities

- ensure that the public sector respects the rights of persons with Disabilities

- ensure that the private sector and individuals respect the rights of persons with Disabilities

- undertake research and development of accessible goods, services, and technology for persons with Disabilities and encourage others to undertake such research

- provide accessible information about assistive technology to persons with Disabilities

- promote training on the rights of the convention to professionals and staff who work with persons with Disabilities

- consult with and involve persons with Disabilities in developing and implementing legislation and policies and in decision-making processes that concern them.

States are expected to achieve this through national frameworks that 'promote, protect, and monitor'. The specific rights identify the existing civil, cultural, economic, political, and social human rights, affirming that persons with Disabilities also hold those rights.

The enabling measures identify specific steps that states must take to ensure an enabling environment for the enjoyment of human rights, namely: awareness-raising, ensuring accessibility, ensuring protection and safety in situations of risk and humanitarian emergencies, promoting access to justice, ensuring personal mobility, enabling habilitation and rehabilitation, and collecting statistics and data.

The National Disability Strategy

From a policy side of things, we also have something called the National Disability Strategy, which 'sees departments and agencies in every corner of Government setting out how they will do their bit to bring about the practical and lasting change that will make a material difference to the lives of Disabled people right across our country' (UK Parliament, 2023b). The National Disability Strategy takes all the laws we have, identifies the areas we need to improve on such as education or social care, and creates a commitment by the Government to address these areas, break down barriers, and increase the equality of opportunity and participation.

For example, the 2021 National Disability Strategy says 'ensure fairness and equality – empower(ing) Disabled people by promoting fairness and equality of opportunities, outcomes and experiences'.

The strategies which the Government delivers are to create a platform for the long-term ambitions 'to put Disabled people at the heart of Government policy and service delivery'. Effectively they set out the plans for the future to address the ableism that we have. We think it is really important to say here that these strategies have received very mixed feedback over the years on their design and whether they have fulfilled the promises or not, with the strategies themselves saying that the Government must demonstrate that they are 'following through on these dedications'.

With that aside, however, it is yet another demonstration of how policy can have an effect on smashing down ableism. Policy doesn't just have to be from the Government, far from it. All organisations, charities, and groups across all sectors have internal policies on how they operate and they should all include sections on diversity, equity, and inclusion, which also refer to Disability.

By creating these policies we are effectively setting rules of behaviour and action for how we behave while at work and as leaders. A violation of these rules results in repercussions – so what do we have here? Another great key to abolishing and unlearning ableism.

Physical accessibility in design

As we are all learning by now, one of the biggest barriers that Disabled people face is physical accessibility, and how the lack of accessibility in the built environment is heavily influencing the existence of ableism. Did you know that UK building regulations play a role in this? Our building regulations actually set out the 'minimum expectations for designing, building, extension and amendment of any new or existing buildings within the UK', and that it is actually compulsory to adhere to these (Historic England, 2024). Any new building that is built has to adhere to minimum standards of safety and accessibility if for public use, and the designs have to be pre-approved before they can be built.

For example:

- **Entrances:** Buildings should have at least one accessible entrance, ideally the main entrance. The entrance should be wide enough for wheelchair users, and the approach route should be safe and convenient.

- **Doorways:** Should have a clear opening width of at least 775 mm.

- **Corridors:** Should be wide enough for wheelchair users to navigate and turn.

- **Ramps:** Should have a gradient of no more than 1:12, a width of at least 1500 mm, and landing areas at the top and bottom.

Getting really technical and down to the detail now, there is a very long document called *Access to and use of buildings: Approved Document M*. British Standards (if we're getting fancy, *BS 8300 Design of an accessible and inclusive built environment. Buildings – code of practice*) enhance Document M to say how accessibility is included where correct and necessary, and basically the two work together (UK Government, 2015).

This means that we do have legal grounds to challenge a building that fails to be accessible to us, and anyone creating a new building has to think about Disabled people at the point of design – is this ableism through lack of accessibility banished? Well, unfortunately at the moment there is a small loophole, and when we say small, we mean big.

Document M can annoyingly be overridden, for example if the building is listed and temporary solutions can be built instead, which may not be fully accessible. The other contributor to this very large loophole is 'minimum standards of accessibility'. Yuck, what a phrase. Minimum standards *should* mean that every single aspect of accessibility is considered and included. Minimum should mean maximum. Because of this loophole, we all need to encourage the meaning of 'minimum standards of accessibility' to be raised, and by unlearning this form of ableism which is our law, we can encourage planners, designers, and builders to think more about Disabled people. In spite of this loophole, because of the Equality Act and PSED and everything else we have spoken about, Disabled people do have the right to hold a lack of physical accessibility to account.

Deep breaths, there's still a bit more to cover (chunky one this, isn't it?).

Code of conduct

Something that you might not think to be relevant but is, surprisingly, is a very specific piece of policy: The Members of Parliament (MP) (the people we vote for at a General Election and who sit in the House of Commons) Code of Conduct. This MP Code of Conduct sets out how our policy leaders are expected to behave while in their position. It guides their behaviour, ethics, and the attitudes that they hold. Specifically relating to our conversation of ableism, before you all wonder where on earth we are going with this, our MPs have a 'duty to uphold the law, including the general law against discrimination' (UK Parliament, 1995). In other words, the people who make, design, and pass our laws have to make sure they are tackling ableism head on and not behaving in a way which encourages Disabled people to be treated less favourably.

Now the importance of Disabled representation and consultation is a whole other conversation which we will be exploring within Chapter 10 on representation, but important to note here is yet another piece of policy whereby Disabled people should be protected from discrimination and be able to hold our leaders to account.

Earlier in this chapter, we explored the definition of Disability, and how it encompasses a broad range of conditions. It is important to therefore note the Mental Health Act of 1983, which sets out and protects the rights of those detained for their safety, enhances the definitions of the Equality Act for those with mental health conditions, and lays down the right to care and treatment. Our entire benefit, social, and welfare system also fits in here as a policy which is (theoretically) designed to prevent the discrimination of Disabled people, with Employment Support Allowance and Personal Independence Payments.

There are also lots of other pieces of legislation that are specifically designed for particular conditions and Disabilities such as the incoming Down Syndrome Act, the Rare Diseases Act, The Police and Criminal Evidence Act (which sets out your rights as a Disabled person dealing with the police), and the Children's Act. All of these again provide further protections for Disabled rights and take steps towards the removal of ableism from our society and governing laws.

Phew, we've made it to the end.

As we have explored in this chapter, there is an extensive framework of policy, legislation, and protected Disability rights aimed at the removal and prevention of ableism. And it isn't just the UK – countries around the world are more and more adopting Disability-specific and anti-discrimination laws, and, as we've learned, are actually coming together as a united task force to create laws that bind us all together to create consistency of rights.

It is very easy at this point to say, well clearly it isn't working, what is the point, why are we experiencing ableism everywhere if it is illegal to discriminate against Disabled people? And this question is 100 percent valid and needs to be answered. Why are we? As we learned from the Disability history chapter, our negative attitudes and treatment of Disabled people are so deeply entrenched within our biases that we have a long way to go to unlearn this behaviour. But what we do know from this chapter is that the expectations of behaviour are set, we know what we are legally bound to do, and importantly we know as Disabled people what we are entitled to, our rights, and the right to defend ourselves and create accountability. We have come a long way already from the days of asylums, workhouses, and old legislation like the Poor Law, the Lunacy Act, and the Equality Act of 2006, but that doesn't mean we should rest on our laurels. We need to increase the pace of progress and look at how we can ensure that our policies and laws are actively anti-ableist.

CHAPTER 9

Unlearning Ableism:
Accessibility

> Disability and inaccessibility are a package deal. You are born or acquire Disability and then boom...you have signed up to a lifetime of disabling, inaccessible barriers. Oh what joy it is to navigate a society not designed for you... And when you design without accessibility in mind, you are designing to exclude. You are contributing to this exclusion.

From the moment they get up to the moment they go to bed, Disabled people experience one inaccessible barrier after another. That is what it means to be Disabled by society. That is what it means to navigate a society that has not been designed for you. Sometimes, a person will know in advance that they're going to face inaccessible barriers, giving them time to plan and prepare. But most of the time inaccessibility is thrust on a person, appearing as:

- inaccessible signage
- no accessible entrances to buildings
- restricted public transport
- no accessible restrooms or toilets
- accessible spaces that are being used as additional storage places

- unusable websites, products, or services
- poor contrasted or small font menus
- inaccessible ways to communicate with a company.

This list is far from exhaustive.

Inaccessibility is everywhere and anywhere

There is no running from it, no hiding from it, and when confronted with it, Disabled people are faced with a choice. Do I speak up, and say this is inaccessible? Or do I say nothing, and just mask my way through this?

If and when we do speak up, our needs are often labelled or viewed as special, extra, or additional. It's as if no one has individual needs, as if Disabled people's access needs are them asking for too much, or it's them being dramatic, needy, or some other misguided ableist belief. Yes, even when we do speak up, we experience situations that mean we have to advocate that much more, have to speak up that much more, have to ask to be included that much more. Disabled people's needs are needs, just like anyone else's.

Everyone has needs. Needs are human. But unlike non-Disabled people's needs, some Disabled people have access needs. They might need an accessible way to engage with a product or service, they might need an adjustment or accommodation to do their job, but that doesn't make their needs any more special than anyone else's, nor does it make a Disabled person any less capable. If Disabled people's needs are so special, surely we shouldn't be still having to challenge the inaccessible and advocating for accessible change? If Disabled people's needs are so special, surely they would be fulfilled without the need to ask?

As a society, we rarely think about Disabled people when we design an environment, website, product, or service. This isn't done out of malice, but most of us are blissfully unaware that we are even creating inaccessible barriers or adding to existing ones. Unless a person has lived experience of Disability or has proximity to Disability, it's likely that they will have come across the word 'accessibility' but mistakenly believed it to be only about lifts and ramps or about how someone accesses a building. In doing so, they fail to realise the significant role accessibility plays in a Disabled person's life, and how by taking the time to make a website or product accessible we are helping to reduce inaccessible barriers, the umpteenth inaccessible barrier that person has experienced that day.

'But it's something for Disabled people to have to worry about'

Make no mistake, accessibility is not a 'Disability problem,' it is an 'everyone problem'. It is a problem for our future selves when we inevitably experience permanent or temporary Disability, and if not us, then someone close to us. It is an organisation problem when they can't attract Disabled customers, candidates, clients, or if they find themselves in hot water due to failing to meet legal requirements. It is an education problem when they fail to create environments for Disabled young people to succeed.

Accessibility is an everyone problem because every single day, each of us, either Disabled or non-Disabled, benefit from accessibility at work, in our homes, in our communities. For example, when we:

- use a voice assistant on our phones, laptops, or home devices, such as Siri, Alexa, or Bixby
- use the voice on our GPS sat navs

- use an electric toothbrush
- use a lift or automated doors
- listen to an audio book or read captions on a movie
- use remote controls
- use heated blankets
- wear Velcro clothing.

Each of these products was designed for Disabled people but is now used and enjoyed by everyone. That is *universal design* – where products are designed to support Disabled people but can universally benefit others.

When we talk about accessibility benefitting everyone, we are talking about universal design. But sadly, we are not provided with the opportunities or resources to learn about accessibility or universal design, not in school, not in education, and not in our everyday lives. But a word of caution: there is no end destination to accessibility, and principles of universal design are great but will not be the final answer.

So, what is accessibility?

Spoiler, accessibility is not just about lifts and ramps; it goes beyond physical access. Accessibility is about designing and creating environments, experiences, products, and services which can be used by as many people as possible. It includes:

- digital accessibility
- physical accessibility
- communication accessibility
- educational accessibility
- healthcare accessibility
- transportation accessibility
- employment accessibility.

Accessibility is not one thing, but rather it is about removing the barriers that disable people across every part of our society. It is removing these barriers and ensuring that Disabled people have equitable opportunities to engage with, participate in, and experience life.

Imagine spending every day being made to bounce a ball back and forth against a wall but every day new barriers and obstacles appear preventing you from being able to throw the ball at the wall. At the start of the day, you are frustrated and annoyed at these barriers, but sometimes you find ways around them; towards the end of the day, you may have managed to overcome them all or just a few. However, the next day, the barriers are different. They are ever-present and ever-changing, preventing you from further progressing. This is what it is to experience inaccessibility. You find a way around one inaccessible barrier and whoops, there's another ready to take its place.

Equality vs equity

At its core accessibility is equity. Not equality but equity. We make this distinction as people often confuse equality and equity.

Equality is about treating everyone equally. It means giving everyone the chance to apply for a job, access a store, join a group. Equality is saying we have this job, and we are posting it, everyone is welcome to apply.

Equity goes a step further by ensuring that an individual's needs and circumstances are taken into consideration. Equity recognises that we do not all have the same privilege, power, circumstances, or experiences. We do not all start from the same position in life.

Whereas equality is saying there is a job and everyone is welcome to apply, to make this equitable you would create a universally accessible recruitment process and offer people adjustments and accommodations should they need.

Imagine when you purchased this book you were given a free pair of shoes. In fact, when anyone purchases this book, they are given a free pair of shoes. We are giving everyone a pair of shoes – sounds equal, right? Slight problem, however: every pair of shoes we are giving away are a UK size ten. This means these shoes aren't going to fit everyone. We also have to take into consideration that some people prefer certain shoes over another pair, some people feel more comfortable not to wear any, and some people cannot wear shoes at all. So, what started as us trying to treat everyone equally, failed to take into account each individual's circumstances.

Equity addresses this. Equity would be us asking each individual when purchasing the book which pair of shoes they would like, what size they need, or if there is a shoe alternative that would work better for them. We have moved from equality to equity. We now are treating everyone equally and we are also recognising their individual needs and circumstances. Accessibility is creating an equitable experience. Accessibility is taking into account that not everyone accesses or engages with things in the same way.

Whether it is an environment you are building, a product you are creating, or a service you are selling, accessibility should always be part of the design and creation process. When it is not, you have missed a step in the process, or rather the process is incomplete. When accessibility is at the core of your design, you are favouring more than non-Disabled people. You are eliminating the barriers that prevent Disabled people from being included.

Accessibility can mean different things to an individual

If you were to ask one Disabled person what an accessible working environment looks like for them, one person might say they require a brightly lit space, whereas another might say they need a dimly lit space. If you ask a person their preferred communication style, one person might request written communication, another verbal, or another sign language. What accessibility looks like for one person can differ for another, and sometimes what is accessible to one person is not always accessible for them at another time. Some people might find it easier to read dark text on a white background, whereas others might prefer dark text on a pastel background because the white is inaccessible for them.

Accessibility is not the destination but rather it is working to make the journey as smooth as possible for as many people as possible. It is recognising that we all access things in different ways; it is working to provide alternative ways to engage and access. It is designing for the many instead of for the few.

Accessibility and ableism – the barrier-riddled frontier

When we consider the current definition of ableism, 'the less favourable treatment of Disabled people', it is clear that inaccessibility is a form of ableism. Ableism is oppression; it stops Disabled people from engaging, participating, and experiencing. Inaccessibility stops Disabled people from being included. It hinders their engagement and participation across society. It stops them from entering the workplace, accessing goods and services, from attending events, right down to being able to understand and perceive information.

Accessibility is not a one-size-fits-all concept, but rather it is designing to be as inclusive as possible. To do this we must be universally designing things to be accessible. Universal design means designing for everyone, rather than viewing accessibility as an afterthought, a nice to have or something additional to add. The philosophy of universal design is to make products, services, environments, experiences, and systems as usable to as many people, regardless of Disability or age, from the get-go.

For example, an organisation's website is inaccessible, so rather than make it accessible by hiring someone to fix it, they may decide to use an accessibility toolbar/overlay/widget. Let's just call them overlays for now. Overlays appear on top of a webpage. They provide a user with tools enabling them to make surface-level changes to a webpage or website (font, sizing, contrast etc.).

They do not, however, write alt text for images (a way to make images accessible for screen readers), they do not fix the reading order of a page (how you navigate a webpage), they do not fix broken links (links on a webpage that are unclear and don't tell a user where it takes them should they click it). These overlays, although sold as a solution to make websites fully accessible, do not actually do so. They have been known to create issues for Disabled users, interfering with a user's own assistive technology, and causing unpredictable behaviours. Website overlays do not make a website accessible. In fact, in the last few years in the US there have been a significant number of accessibility lawsuits against organisations who have been using accessibility overlays as a substitute for universally designed websites.

We should also point out that there is a difference between usability and accessibility. Usability focuses on ensuring that a user has a great experience and that they can interact with digital products and services in an easy efficient way, whereas accessibility focuses on the experiences of Disabled people, ensuring that Disabled people can engage and use the same products and services.

Accessibility is a shared responsibility

We all have a responsibility to take accountability for accessibility. It is not down to Disabled people alone to advocate for accessibility. Each of us contributes to inaccessible barriers, therefore it is up to all of us to make change, to make accessible change.

Before we look at the ways you can unlearn the ableism in the way you design, build, create, and communicate, let's debunk some myths about accessibility.

Myth	Truth
'Accessibility is for Disabled people'	We all benefit from accessibility. Just look around your home and you will find that a lot of products you benefit from using were created specifically for Disabled people.
'Accessibility does not impact me'	It is not 'if' you become Disabled, it is when you experience Disability, and if not you, it will be someone you know.
'Accessibility is a trend, nice to have.'	Accessibility has never been a trend or nice to have. In fact, within the US already and in Europe, accessibility is a legal requirement for organisations.
'Accessibility means my product or service won't be as aesthetically pleasing'	We do not have to compromise design to make something accessible. Accessibility and aesthetics can go hand in hand. Accessible design can be fresh, fun, vibrant, and sexy.

cont.

Myth	Truth
'Accessibility only applies to websites'	Accessibility applies to environments, products, services, processes, workplaces, education, transport, healthcare – need we go on?
'Adjustments/ accommodations resolve inaccessibility'	Adjustments/accommodations do not fix poor design. They are tools that support a user, but they do not magically fix an inaccessible website, process, or building.
'Accessibility is about compliance'	Accessibility is about providing equal and equitable access to products, services, environments, and so on. While there are more and more regions making accessibility a legal compliance, that does not make it just a compliance issue.
'Accessibility is the answer'	Accessibility is not the answer; it is one step in the process of ensuring that environments, workplaces, events, processes, and so on are usable by as many people as possible.
'Accessibility is a one-time thing'	Accessibility should be continuously monitored, tested, and reviewed. Technology evolves, and so does the way we engage with services, products, and goods. We should always be striving to continuously improve.

Accessibility is expensive

If you have learned anything about us reading this book you will know that we like to be upfront and honest with our sharing. We left this example out of the table above because there is a truth and a myth within the statement that accessibility is expensive.

The myth that accessibility is expensive is a narrative that is pushed around businesses to avoid them making any kind of accessible change. Businesses measure effectiveness through return of investment, and the inherent ableism in our society stops us from seeing the value of accessibility.

Organisations fail to understand the return for investment when it comes to accessibility, despite the many studies showing that actually accessibility is a business case, and there is a return for investment.

A report by Accenture, in partnership with Disability:IN and the American Association of People with Disabilities (2018), revealed that companies leading in Disability inclusion reported 28% higher revenue, double the net income, and 30% higher profit margins compared to their peers. These are companies that are taking action to create an accessible, inclusive workplace, and are now enjoying the return for this investment in an accessible, inclusive workplace.

A UK report by Click-Away Pound (Williams & Brownlow, 2016) revealed that 71% of Disabled users will click away from a website if it is inaccessible. The same report also identified that 82% of Disabled customers would spend more money if websites were accessible. In the UK alone, the spending power of Disabled people is estimated at £274 billion annually (Scope, n.d.a) and globally it is $13 trillion dollars (World Economic Forum, 2023). Surely from a consumer point of view this is a market companies need and should be diving into?

Now we aren't mathematicians, but the maths is not adding up. Do you see how frustrating it can sound when a company talks about accessibility being an expense but fails to see that the return for investment goes beyond just capital gain? There are also lots of free things that organisations can do to begin taking accountability for accessibility today and creating a more inclusive workplace, but you will have to keep reading as we explore some of these below and in Chapter 12, Unlearning Ableism: Recruitment and Workplaces.

So, while some companies will no doubt play off accessibility as an expensive investment with no real return, it's up to us to remind them of the above. We need to remind them that change doesn't happen overnight; they need to work with their budgets, and with Disability consultants, and map out what they can do now, and in three months, six months, a year, and so on. Call it an accessibility roadmap.

We did say there is a myth and a truth to the accessibility being expensive

The truth is that for many Disabled people, accessibility is not cheap, and often there is limited or lack of grants or support available. Purchasing equipment to provide support at home, aids, adjustment, assistive technology or having alterations made to the home, car, and so on, does bring an additional expense.

Being Disabled comes with a hidden price tag, which we will explore later in our economics chapter. These additional costs mean that our disposable income isn't always readily available to make adaptions to a new bed, or to fork out a couple of thousand pounds or dollars for a new wheelchair because our own has been damaged. Accessibility often comes with a steep price tag, one which ultimately makes accessibility an unaffordable reality.

The steep costs associated with accessibility are often due to a lack of mass production and investment. Accessibility and assistive technologies are viewed as niche markets, which creates higher production costs per unit. In turn, this has made innovation in this field much slower than other markets, but with the rise of artificial intelligence (AI) and machine learning, who knows what the future holds? Perhaps robots one day will be able to support with accessibility at home, in work, and across society?

But one thing is for sure, accessibility can be expensive for an individual and if we are ever to unlearn the ableism in our society, Disabled people need to be supported to live barrier-free lives which should not cost more simply because we are Disabled.

When accessibility is not part of the process when designing it can be that Disabled people are no longer viewed as potential candidates, clients, customers, or end users. And due to this, businesses fail to recognise the significant market value of the purple pound – that is, the spending power of Disabled people globally.

Designing accessibly isn't about doing the right thing. The right thing is not the same for everyone. Darth Vader thought the right thing to do was wipe out the Jedi, but if you asked another person, they might tell you that wasn't the right thing. So, each person's interpretation of the right thing is different. Therefore, designing accessibly and communicating accessibly isn't the right thing to do; it is the equitable thing to do. It is the inclusive thing to do. It is the anti-ableist thing to do.

Accessibility is not one thing

Accessibility touches and impacts many parts of a Disabled person's life. It can stop us from applying for a job, from engaging with marketing, from attending events, from accessing transport, from being included across society. So, what are some of the forms of accessibility you need to be aware of?

Physical accessibility

When a person hears the word accessibility they tend to think of physical accessibility. We are not saying they are getting it right, or they know it all, but when someone thinks of a lift or ramp, they are thinking of physical access, so they are on the right path. They just haven't considered the bends and junctions in that path. Physical accessibility refers to making built environments accessible for Disabled people, and this includes things like buildings, infrastructure, and public spaces. Think of homes, transport hubs, public sidewalks, offices, restrooms, signage, roads and so on.

Imagine you are trying to find a home and you are Disabled; let's say you are a wheelchair user. Think of that home.

Have you considered that you will likely need wider doorways? This means either finding a home with wider doors or making costly adjustments/accommodations to the existing doorways to widen them.

What about the front door? Does it have steps? Will you need a ramp? If you plan to view this house and it does not have a ramp, how will you even view it? That's a cost to install if it doesn't.

What about the type of house you are viewing? Have you thought about the need for a bungalow rather than a one-story or multi-story house which has stairs? Is there a stair lift to help get you to the top floor if it is not a bungalow? That's potentially another cost you're going to have to consider.

What about the kitchen? Are you able to stand for short periods to use the countertops or have the counter tops been adapted to be low enough to use from your chair? If those counters aren't low enough that's another cost.

We haven't even found a house yet and already the list of suitable homes has dwindled because, surprise, as a society we don't design enough accessible homes for Disabled people.

A study from Inclusion London (2025) found that only 3% of new homes approved in London were suitable for Disabled people. Furthermore, less than 1% were designed specifically for wheelchair users. When we consider that there are 1.2 million wheelchair users in the UK (Atkins Jacob, 2022), it means that wheelchair users have a 1% chance of finding an accessible home. In the US, a report found that less than 5% of American homes are accessible for Disabled people (Real Estate Investor Pulse, 2023) despite there being approximately 5.5 million Americans who use a wheelchair (US Department of Transportation, 2024a), meaning wheelchair users in the US have a 1 in 20 chance of finding an accessible home.

We cannot say there is no demand for accessible homes – the numbers speak for themselves, we are also an aging population, and accessible homes don't just support and benefit Disabled people, but many older people too.

By now you will be starting to understand the multitude of questions a Disabled person must ask themselves before even thinking about renting or buying a home, questions that non-Disabled people would never have to consider. To a wheelchair user and for many Disabled people, an accessible home can feel like a pipe dream, and it isn't just homes. It's public buildings, courthouses, private and public spaces – there are inaccessible physical barriers right across our society, ableist barriers that restrict Disabled people's participation, freedoms, and movements.

> 66 Our built environment is not neutral – it either enables or disables. Architecture reflects society's values, and for too long, it has communicated a clear message: Disabled people are an

afterthought, if considered at all. Stairs, narrow corridors, heavy doors, inaccessible transport – these are not just inconveniences, but manifestations of systemic exclusion.

The problem isn't that Disabled people exist; the problem is that our spaces were not designed with us in mind. This is why user-led design isn't enough – design must be done by us, not just for us. The phrase 'nothing about us without us' must extend beyond policy and into the physical world we all navigate. If exclusion was built in, then it can be designed out again.

Current building regulations and accessibility standards set a low bar, often treating Disability as a box-ticking exercise rather than a fundamental design principle. 'Reasonable adjustments' place the burden on individuals to demand access rather than requiring society to provide it by default. But access is not an add-on – it is a right.

We must shift the narrative from retro-fitted compromises to proactive, inclusive design. This means embedding accessibility into every stage of the design process, ensuring that Disabled designers have a seat at the table, and recognising that Disability is not a niche issue but an inevitable part of human diversity. The built environment can liberate or constrain, empower or exclude. The choice is ours – and it's time to redesign a world where everyone belongs. 99

– Amy Francis-Smith, Royal Institute of British Architects, senior architect and accessible design specialist

Transportation accessibility

This refers to making transport accessible for Disabled people, whether this is public transport, airlines, taxis, private transport companies, and so on. For many Disabled people, leaving the house can feel like a military operation.

- How do I get from point A to point B?
- How accessible is this journey going to be?
- Can I get a taxi?
- Will they refuse my service animal?
- Will they have space for my mobility aid?
- What about the train or bus?
- Will there be access to the station and support to get on and off at stations?
- What do I do if someone has put their pram in the Disabled assigned seating?

These questions are ones Disabled people have to ask before planning any kind of journey. There was an 18% increase of passenger assistance requests from the previous year (Office of Rail and Road, 2025). That's nearly a 20% increase of people having to ask for help when using public transport – where is the independence in that? We should not have to ask for support to be able to travel independently, and while getting this support is often a necessity, it shouldn't mean having to check if a train station is accessible or worrying about being able to get onto the bus, train, or even a flight.

Talking of flying, you have been under a rock if you haven't read the horror stories in the papers about Disabled people and airlines, and the shamefully inhumane treatment of Disabled people while flying. There are stories of Disabled people's wheelchairs being damaged or destroyed, Disabled people dragging themselves up the aisle of the plane to get to the bathroom. The inaccessibility and ableism start from the moment we get to the airport, and continue on the flight, and until the moment we land and leave the airport.

In 2023, the US Department of Transportation received 2685

Disability-related complaints, marking a 28% increase from the 2100 complaints in 2022 (US Department of Transportation, 2024b). When we think of airports we think of a busy loud environment, which for many Disabled people is an obstacle course riddled with barriers. The Royal National Institute of Blind People (2022) found that 43% of passengers with visual impairments reported difficulties with airport signage and navigation. For autistic people, travelling can lead to sensory overload and anxiety and can create difficulties when trying to communicate needs (National Autistic Society, 2025).

Travelling as a Disabled person is a unique experience each time we leave the house. There is no unified approach across airports or airlines, trains, buses, there is no one universal training, but there is hope.

66 Travel is so often seen as something everyone should aspire to, broadening your horizons, and discovering the world. But for Disabled people, the reality is far more complicated. Every trip comes with layers of planning, uncertainty, and often, a quiet calculation of how much we're willing to tolerate just to get from A to B.

It's not just about physical access, though that's still a huge issue. It's cultural. The way staff talk to us (or don't). The assumptions made at airports, at hotels, on transport. The sense that we're not really supposed to be there, or that if we are, we should be grateful. There's still this deep-rooted idea that travel is for the non-Disabled, and if we're part of it, it's either an inspiration story or an inconvenience.

Unlearning ableism means shifting that whole narrative. It's about recognising that access isn't an add-on; it's a fundamental. Culturally, we need to normalise Disabled people being everywhere: on beaches, in cities, at festivals, in hostels, in first class. Not just featured when there's a 'Disability special', but built into the everyday.

We deserve more than to simply 'make do'. We deserve spontaneity, ease, and joy. We deserve to exist in the world without it becoming a fight every time we want to move through it. **99**

– Carrie-Ann Lightley, freelance writer, speaker, and accessible travel specialist

Organisations like the Hidden Disabilities Sunflower work tirelessly across the globe to support Disabled people when travelling, delivering training and providing a sunflower lanyard to wear which can and should be recognised by staff at airports, train stations and so on, making it easier to ask for support. Disabled travellers deserve an equitable, independent experience and the same freedoms as everyone else when travelling.

Educational accessibility

This refers to the inaccessible barriers preventing Disabled people from receiving an equitable education. It is removing barriers so that young Disabled people can gain an education which they understand, in which they can learn, and which is accessible for them. Reports in the UK show that disparities in outcomes between Disabled pupils and their peers are continuing to widen. For 11- and 16-year-olds, the gaps are the widest in over a decade (National Education Union, 2024). We will explore this in more detail in our education chapter.

Health and social care accessibility

This refers to ensuring that Disabled people have access to the medical services, support, and community resources they need to lead independent, fulfilling lives. This means having access to healthcare assistants and access to the assistive technology many of us need to engage and interact with the world – such as walking aids, hearing aids, wheelchairs, and screen readers. It is ensuring that Disabled people have access to diagnosis and treatment and are able to access these resources and supports in accessible and affordable ways. If there is one sector that should understand Disabled people's needs better than others, you would think it would be the healthcare system. Sadly, you would be mistaken.

Imagine you are waiting for the results of a test from the doctor, and you have asked the doctor to call you as a first point of contact, or if they have no other choice but to contact you via writing, you said that you require a larger font. Rather than calling you as per your access need, they send you a letter, in a size 12 font and actually inaccessible to you. Or imagine you are sat in a doctor's office and the doctor is calling patients verbally. What do you do if you are a d/Deaf person who is unable to hear this verbal cue? These things are not rare instances but daily challenges for many Disabled people.

The World Health Organization and United Nations Children's Fund (UNICEF) (2022) reported that over 2.5 billion people need one or more assistive technology aid such as wheelchairs, hearing aids, and communication devices. Despite this, nearly 1 billion people are denied access, especially in low- and middle-income countries where access can be as low as 3%. When access to assistive technology is denied or a person is restricted in the very thing that healthcare should be providing, independence and improving their quality of life become unattainable goals for that Disabled person.

Without assistive technology, some Disabled people will experience barriers communicating their experiences, increase risk to injury, acquire preventable health complications, or face isolation, which in turn may lead to anxiety or depression. The excessive costs of assistive devices and Disability-specific services can make healthcare inaccessible for millions of Disabled people. The lack of understanding of Disability and the social model view of Disability can lead many Disabled people to experience barriers to diagnosis, receiving bias or discrimination from healthcare professionals, and, in many cases, lengthy delays or misdiagnosis before getting a correct diagnosis.

Workplace accessibility

This refers to making working environments, systems, tools, practices, and processes accessible for Disabled people. It is removing the barriers preventing Disabled people from opportunities, participation, and belonging in the workplace. A global survey by Deloitte (2024) found that nearly 90% of Disabled respondents, and people with chronic health conditions or neurodivergence, disclosed their condition to someone at work.

However, only 25% requested workplace adjustments/ accommodations, and 74% had at least one adjustment/ accommodation request denied. Additionally, 60% of respondents were unable to attend work-related events due to accessibility challenges (Deloitte, 2024). Inaccessible barriers in the workplace are present from the moment someone visits a company's website, to the application stage, offer stage, and during employment. We will learn more about ableism and inaccessibility in Chapter 12 on recruitment and workplaces.

Emergency accessibility

This refers to ensuring that Disabled people can access and utilise emergency services during natural disasters, medical emergencies, fires, or evacuations. It includes ensuring that Disabled people can be evacuated if there is a fire in the workplace. It also means ensuring that Disabled people can evacuate during times of war, which, unfortunately, once seemed like a thing from history books past, but now today remains a stark reality. It means ensuring that people can accessibly evacuate, communicate, and engage with services.

According to the United Nations Office for Disaster Risk Reduction, only 25% of Disabled people can evacuate without difficulty during disasters (as cited in ReliefWeb, 2024). More recently during the disastrous fires around Los Angeles in January 2025, CNN News (Mazzeo, 2025) reported that Disabled people were unable to evacuate due to inaccessible transportation and shelters.

When we talk about emergency accessibility, we also have to understand and address the ableist and inaccessible treatment that Disabled people can experience. Instances where law enforcement offices misinterpret behaviours displayed by Disabled people, such as not receiving clear instructions, can lead to escalated responses, including the use of force. Disabled people deserve the same level of safety, care, and protection as non-Disabled people, and misinterpretation often stems from a lack of training and awareness.

These examples of accessibility are not exhaustive.

By now you are realising that there are many different types of accessibility, and you might also be thinking that unless you are in a position of power, you can't make many changes to how society builds that new train station, and you don't create evacuation plans, so what exactly can you do?

We are now going to explore two forms of accessibility, digital and communication accessibility, and it is these two forms of accessibility that we feel everyone should begin to understand and learn about. You will find lots of tips to help you begin to unlearn the ableism that lies within inaccessibility.

Digital and communication accessibility

Digital accessibility

According to a study by WebAIM (2025), 94.8% of the world's top one million websites' home pages have at least one detected Web Content Accessibility Guidelines 2 failure. That means that less than 5% of webpages are fully accessible for Disabled people. Let that sink in.

Imagine trying to apply for a job, but you can't because the webpage is not accessible. Trying to find a service, trying to shop, browse, doom scroll, but you can't because the webpages are not accessible. This is the current state of digital accessibility. It is not inclusive, it is not universally designed, and it is not usable for a lot of Disabled people when:

- an individual posts content on social media
- an organisation shares marketing
- someone builds a webpage
- someone sends a PDF file
- someone shares a graphic for their amazing inclusive event.

The likelihood is they have done these things without making them accessible.

For individuals using assistive technology, you will have created barriers unseen to the naked eye. For other users, it might be overwhelming, too flashy, poorly contrasted, difficult to navigate or unclear, creating a negative user experience for lots of different Disabled people.

TAB TEST

A quick visit to an organisation's website will tell us if an organisation is as inclusive as it claims to be. In fact, anyone can check the accessibility of a website. There are many free website accessibility checkers online which you can utilise, or you can simply run a tab test.

A tab test is when you use the tab key on the keyboard instead of using a mouse or mousepad to navigate a webpage. Remember, not everyone is able to use a mouse so by using the tab key on your keyboard you are able to experience how a webpage will navigate for them.

1. Open up your chosen organisation's webpage on a desktop.

2. Now using the tab key on your keyboard, tab along.

3. Notice the order of the page content as you tab. Does it move as it should in order? Are you able to navigate menus and content? Or are you jumping all around the page?

This test is a quick way to establish if a page is accessible for a person unable to use a mouse or mousepad. A website visitor should be able to navigate through menus and content in logical order. This is only one test of many, but it is one you can try yourself. You can also use free tools like WAVE's online checker to run a full accessibility check on a website. Creating a fully accessible website takes time, resources, and specialised support, especially if it wasn't designed with accessibility to begin with.

Now, you anti-ableist warrior, let's look at some other ways you can begin taking accountability for digital accessibility.

ADD ALT TEXT TO AN IMAGE
Alt text describes an image online. It is typically embedded into an image, meaning without a screen reader or some kind of overlay, you won't be able to see it with the naked eye. But a person using a

screen reader will have the description read aloud to them, helping them create a mental picture of the image. All digital images should include alt text. That includes images on websites, emails, presentations, slide decks, social media, PDFs, and apps. When writing alt text, ask yourself what the purpose of the image is and then describe it. Keep it short, factual, and, most of all, relevant to the image.

ADD AN IMAGE DESCRIPTION TO AN IMAGE

Not everyone uses a screen reader and not everyone feels comfortable or confident with them. Image description is an alternative way to make an image accessible. Much like alt text, an image description describes an image. While alt text is a short description, an image description can be slightly longer and more detailed. We are not saying you need to point everything out in the image, like the person has a spot on their nose or there is a single strand of grey hair, but rather to include details like colour, texture, and location. Unlike alt text, however, an image description is visible. It should be placed in a caption or a text box beside the image or, if on social media, within the body of the message.

CAPTION VIDEOS

Captions are text-based representation of all spoken words and narration, or relevant sounds within a video. Although originally thought to be used by only d/Deaf/hard of hearing individuals, captions are an example of universal design benefitting everyone. People who are neurodivergent, people who are learning a new language, or someone in a public space who forgets their headphones but wants to watch an episode of something can all benefit from captions.

Captions should match spoken words, and they should always be accessible, meaning they should be readable. There's a trend where organisations and individuals use poor contrasting colours together, making the captions themselves unreadable. Please make sure your captions are accessible, use a clear font, place them at the bottom and middle of the screen, and please always check the colour contrast if opting to move away from black and white. The difference between 'open captions' and 'closed captions' is that open captions are burned into a video, meaning you can't remove them, and closed captions can be switched on or off and are added by the platform the video is uploaded on.

CHECK COLOUR CONTRAST

Colour contrast describes the difference between two colours. Colour contrast ratio is the measurement of that difference. By checking the colour contrast ratio, we are able to identify if text or any visual elements are legible from the background colour. To check the contrast ratio, you will need two things:

- You need the hex codes or RGB values of both the foreground and background colours you are using. (Every colour has its own code to help make it uniquely identifiable; that is what the hex codes or RBG values refer to.)

- You need an online tool like WebAIM's colour contrast checker, or you can use a web extension. This will allow you to input the foreground and background colours to check if they meet Web Content Accessibility Guidelines (WCAG) and can be used accessibly. (More about the WCAG guidelines below.)

LABEL LINKS CORRECTLY

Labels help assistive technology users understand where a link will take them. Most people underestimate the importance of this and use vague labels that don't exactly tell the user where or what they will find by using the link. For example, a link label reading 'click here' doesn't tell a person where they are going. It is like a game of guess where. Give labels appropriate titles. Rather than use 'click here', try describing where the link will take an individual. 'Read more about our DEI initiatives on our DEI page.' Spot the difference?

STOP RELYING ON PDF FILES

Unless you have made a PDF accessible, it won't be. PDFs are not anyone's first choice for accessibility, so instead try opting for open-source documents, like Microsoft Word.

By utilising Microsoft products, you can take advantage of the in-built accessibility checker, which reviews and provides guidance on creating accessible Microsoft files. Unless you have a person or team making your PDFs accessible, the likelihood is they aren't accessible. So please stop using them until you can do this.

ADD AN ACCESSIBILITY STATEMENT

An accessibility statement should be visible on the footer of a website. It provides a user with information about the current state of accessibility on your website. It gives details of your current accessibility level, any flagged issues or work you are currently undergoing, and it should also provide a point of contact with alternative ways to reach out in case a user experiences any issues. This statement is about showing intent. It's not a disclaimer to get away with not fixing your website, rather the opposite. It highlights that you are a company/individual that is holding itself accountable to a standard of accessibility, a standard of anti-ableist inclusion.

DON'T USE WEBSITE OVERLAYS

We know we have already covered website overlays, but please don't fall into the trap. Don't let an overlay company sell you the promise of an accessible website; don't get sold on a lie.

Of course, no one is expected to suddenly be an expert of accessibility with just a few tips and a bit of background information, and that is where the Web Content Accessibility Guidelines come in. The guidelines are created and managed by the World Wide Web Consortium (W3C) and provide a detailed framework on how to create accessible content online. These standards are recognised globally and should be adhered to.

To learn more about the Web Content Accessibility Guidelines and the various levels of accessibility (A, AA, AAA) visit www.w3.org. We all have to take accountability for creating accessible, equitable experiences online. We all have to take ownership and be open to learning. Continue learning by utilising free resources like www.accessible-social.com, by Alexa Heinrich, which helps individuals learn how to create accessible content online.

Communication accessibility

People take for granted the diverse needs and preferences individuals might have when it comes to communicating. They don't consider these needs and preferences because they are so accustomed to communicating to one group of people, non-Disabled people. By being proactive and embodying inclusive actions you can begin to communicate in a much more universally accessible way. But remember, you still need to always ask a person their preferred communication style; you cannot assume. Below you will find some accessible tips to support you when communicating, tips that can be used in your personal and professional life.

USE CLEAR STRAIGHTFORWARD LANGUAGE

Use clear and straightforward language in both verbal and written communication. Don't overcomplicate things by using jargon or acronyms, unless you are actually going to explain what they mean. If you haven't ever heard a screen reader reading acronyms, trust us, you would not enjoy it. Want to try to download a free screen reader like Google Chrome or try the screen reader that's built into your phone's accessibility? If you must use an acronym, make sure you tell the reader what it means and for the love of inclusion, try not to use lots and lots of them; it is not fun!

USE SHORTER SENTENCES

It is so easy to switch off when you are being presented with words and words and never-ending words. Break information down into digestible sentences and remember to breathe between each sentence.

PROVIDE CLEAR DIRECTION

Stop relying on people being able to read between the lines. The lines are blurred for some of us. Don't assume people will know what you mean; you need to say it clearly. If you are asking someone to do a task, be clear about what it is you're asking. Asking someone to, 'Copy this information onto a PowerPoint slide' and then getting angry with them because they didn't spellcheck or condense the information is unfair because you were not clear. The direction given should have been, 'Take this information, spellcheck it, condense it, then put it on a PowerPoint slide.' Clarity matters.

DON'T RELY ON VISUAL AIDS ALONE

Yes, visual aids may work for some but be sure to provide alt text and image descriptions for any visual aids, or if in person, be sure to describe the visual aid being used.

OFFER ALTERNATIVE FORMATS

Offer alternative formats for people to engage in diverse ways. Examples include text, braille, audio, larger font, or easy read versions.

OFFER SIGN LANGUAGE

Provide sign language interpretation for live events, meetings, interviews, video content, gatherings, and so on.

VISUAL DESCRIPTION

Provide a visual description of yourself when presenting, speaking, or training. A visual description is a brief description describing what a speaker looks like. This includes things like what you look like and what you are wearing.

SET AN AGENDA

Before any meetings, interviews, and briefings, send a clear agenda outlining what to expect from the event. This clarity can help someone prepare and come with any questions that they might have.

FOLLOW UP

After any meetings, interviews, and briefings, send follow-up notes detailing any actions required and who is responsible for such actions, things that were discussed, and any reminders or calls to action.

ALWAYS ASK

Always ask a person their preferred communication style and respect it: if we say we prefer verbal communication, we prefer verbal. Be sure to also ask if adjustments and accommodations are needed before any trainings, meetings, interviews, events, and so on.

For many Disabled people, when we have shared our preferred way of communication, we have been dismissed, overlooked, ignored, or in some cases outright rejected. We've been told we don't pay attention, that we ask too many questions, we seem distracted, we need to focus or just try harder. Try harder implies we can and should just get over the barriers we are experiencing when being communicated to in a way which is not accessible for us. Would you ask a blind/visually impaired person to look harder at an image to see it? Would you ask a d/Deaf/hard of hearing person to listen harder as you deliver training? We really hope your answer was no, of course not. But yet for many Disabled people we are told to try harder, despite in many cases having tried as hard as possible.

Inaccessible communication is inaccessible, and no trying on the individual's side will fix that. This kind of response is privilege. It shows a complete disregard for accessibility, and it is a massive middle finger to the Disabled person being told to try harder. No matter how much you try, you cannot force Disabled people to conform to an inaccessible form of communication, or any inaccessible barrier for that matter.

WHAT TO DO IF YOU GET IT WRONG

When someone points out that something is inaccessible don't see it as a personal attack on you, your work, content, event, or wherever the inaccessible barrier lies. See it as an opportunity to gain experience, to improve, to make a change.

A change that won't just benefit one person, but lots of people. Yes, it might feel uncomfortable when this happens, but we have to learn to be comfortable with the uncomfortable. We have to learn to be able to see this for what it is: a person who has experienced numerous inaccessible barriers that day asking to be included. Open yourself up to learning. Create space for people to provide feedback, to ask for accessible change, to share their preferred communication style in a space where everyone can be comfortable and safe to actually say something in the first place.

And remember to include Disabled people

When designing or creating environments, it is paramount that Disabled people are consulted first. Assuming something will be accessible does not make it so. We have seen repeatedly non-Disabled people designing ramps for buildings, thinking it to be the most amazing accessible thing, when had they asked a person using a wheelchair, they would have been advised, 'Well actually, this is too steep.' Or accessible restrooms, spaces that are meant to be designed to accommodate different access needs, but instead do not meet any kind of accessibility requirements or standards. It's all well and good if you added a lift to your building, but if the doors inside aren't wide enough for a wheelchair or other mobility aids, then it's as useful as a lock with no key.

For too long, ableism has allowed inaccessibility to lay the foundations of our exclusion, but we say no more. Inaccessibility. keeps Disabled people oppressed, and, make no mistake, inaccessibility is ableist and we need to get comfortable with calling it that. Inaccessibility is ableist.

By taking accountability for accessibility, you can unlearn the ableism that has prevented you from learning to design to include. By recognising the diverse needs of those around you, you can begin to communicate in ways beyond a non-Disabled, neuro-majority standard. By making accessibility part of the conversation, and part of everyday life, we can create a tomorrow that includes everyone – a tomorrow that is accessible, inclusive, and anti-ableist.

CHAPTER 10
Unlearning Ableism: Representation

> **Representation is one of the most discussed topics of conversation around Disability and ableism, and also arguably one of the most important chapters of this book. Conscious vs unconscious, accidental vs incidental, intentional vs unintentional. When we say representation matters, we really mean it.**

Representation is powerful. From the young Disabled child to the grown Disabled adult, seeing or hearing people who look like you offers hope, connection, and opportunity.

When we look at the typical representation of Disability, we typically see one thing, the symbol of a wheelchair – heck, it's the international symbol of Disability used on car parks, bathrooms, bumper stickers, and websites. Typically, if a wheelchair user is shown they tend to be a white person. Disability is the most diverse minority group in the world, and using a wheelchair does not represent the beautiful diversity of Disability, such as neurodivergence, chronic conditions, limb differences, non-visible Disabilities.

As we learned in our study of Disability history, Disabled people have existed since the dawn of time, so surely that must mean that in society we are quite literally everywhere. When we look at our representation and portrayal, we must also be everywhere, right? Sadly not.

Below are some shocking statistics that help put into perspective the current state of Disabled representation across the world. Keep in mind that Disabled people make up nearly 17% of the global population, as we learned earlier.

- Less than 2% of Members of Parliament in the UK are Disabled (John Smith Centre, 2023)

- None of the FTSE 100 company senior leaders identify as Disabled (Disability:IN, 2023).

- Disabled entrepreneurs hold just 0.1% of the share of conversation in investment (Access2Funding, 2023).

- Only 2.4% of all characters who spoke or had names in the top 100 movies ever made are Disabled (Smith *et al.*, 2016).

- Only 1.6% of daytime TV shows feature a Disabled character (Disability Horizons, 2022).

- Only 4.1% of watchable media features Disability themes (Nielsen, 2022).

- Total screen time for Disabled people is 8.8% and 0.4% for people with non-visible Disabilities (Nielsen, 2022).

- There is a 29% employment gap between Disabled and non-Disabled adults (Office for National Statistics, 2022b).

- Just 4% of children's books feature Disabled main characters (CCBlogC, 2019).

- The likelihood of a Disabled adult completing higher education is 25% compared to 43% of non-Disabled adults (Office for National Statistics, 2022a).

I mean, we could go on and on and on, filling this whole chapter with statistics like these…

When we say Disabled representation is doing badly, we really mean it.

There is a massive misconception that when we are talking about representation we are only talking about media, things like TV, film, and social media, but it is so much more than this. Representation is about every aspect of life, from business, to fashion, to media, to sports, to leadership to development. Disabled representation is not just about who is in front of our screens; it is also about who is behind them, and both play equal importance. It is about Disabled people not being in positions of power within business, politics, education, and every other aspect of our society.

So now we understand the position of play for Disabled people that we are currently in, let us take a deep dive into unlearning this section of our ableism, by first understanding why, and then how.

Representation is actually defined in two ways, both as a noun and as a verb. As a noun, representation is 'the fact of including all' and as a verb, it is 'where something or someone is presenting on behalf of another something or someone'. Both definitions are equally as important as one another, and both play a part in the conversation of unlearning ableism.

" As a Black Disabled woman, I navigate a world that sometimes overlooks the richness of my identity. Representation holds transformative power, but when confined to narrow narratives, it can perpetuate ableism rather than dismantle it. Frequently, Black Disabled individuals are either invisible in media and leadership or depicted solely through lenses of struggle and adversity. Such portrayals fail to capture our resilience, joy, and significant cultural contributions.

Black and Brown communities often face stigma surrounding Disability, leading to further isolation and lack of support. Authentic representation transcends mere visibility; it encompasses being genuinely heard, valued, and granted the agency to lead. It's about moving beyond narratives of pity or mere perseverance to those highlighting agency and equity. Our stories deserve to be portrayed in their entirety, not just as tales of struggle but as blueprints for a more inclusive society. To unlearn ableism, we must champion representation that mirrors the full spectrum of our identities: bold, multifaceted, and unapologetically authentic. "

– Terri-Louise Brown, Founder and CEO of Talks With MS

The Solar System effect

We are going to give you an analogy to explain the importance of representation, and why a lack of representation is having such a damaging effect on the Disabled community.

Pause and imagine for a moment the sun, a burning, powerful inferno sitting proud and centre in the middle of our Milky Way galaxy. All of the planets in our galaxy were formed from a disk-shaped cloud around the sun, and after their formation, each of these planets have kept spinning around the sun in this cloud, at the same speeds, same distances, and same directions each year (for any science buffs this is called the heliocentric orbit).

The sun remains at the centre of these swirling planets, controlling the gravity which keeps them all in their place, and because the sun is the strongest element of our galaxy nothing else is able to throw the planets off course. The sun symbolises representation, and each of the planets swirling around it represents different sectors of our lives; business, sports, media, politics, fashion, and so on. Representation as the strongest element around holds the power to change the course of each of these planets and is feeding the direction and intention of each of these sectors.

Without better Disabled representation, the ability for our world to change to be more inclusive to Disabled people is significantly halted. Awareness, education, access, opportunity, and participation all stem from representation; everything feeds in and everything feeds out. Without representation in media, we are not destigmatising and raising awareness of Disability; without representation in fashion, we are preventing accessibility in clothing brands; without representation in business and senior leadership, we are halting Disabled employment; without representation within our political leadership, we are preventing inclusive and equitable legislation and policy. If you remember one phrase from this chapter, then it is this: nothing about us without us. Disabled people must be present at the conversation, from the point of design, across all sectors, across all levels of seniority, and that starts with representation.

Why do we need better Disabled representation?

Representation is a catalyst for change. Improving representation is the key for unlearning ableism and moving forward towards equity for Disabled people – let's explore why.

Disabled representation breaks down the stereotypes, the misconceptions, and the presumptions made about Disabled people. What are the first thoughts people jump to when they hear the word Disabled: helplessness, dependence, inability, pity, inspirational. These associations are widely incorrect and harmful. Positive representation shines a spotlight on the real side of Disability: talent, beauty, skill, diversity, creativity, determination, and reliance. It breaks down a significant ableism barrier, and inherent attitudinal misconceptions.

Look at the majority of fashion shows, look in catalogues, look online; there is a glaring lack of Disabled representation in fashion. Only 0.02% of models during major fashion weeks in 2021 were visibly Disabled (de Castro, 2024).

It's as if designers and brands don't think of us as wearing clothes – but trust us, no one wants us all running around in our birthday suits! Clothes can make us feel confident, they can make us feel powerful, they can make us feel sexy, and they should be comfortable. Yet for many Disabled people, finding suitable clothing is not easy. We can't just shop off the rack, or order online, sometimes due to physical barriers to entering stores, or inaccessible websites, but mainly because fashion hasn't considered the diverse needs of Disabled people and fails to create adaptive clothing. This can mean having to buy clothes and then having them altered to make them comfortable. In fact, 75% of Disabled people feel their needs are not met by the fashion industry (Webster, 2025).

> 66 As an adaptive fashion designer, I have seen first-hand how the industry continues to overlook Disabled people, despite the fact that over 20% of the global population has a Disability. Fashion is a fundamental part of self-expression and identity, yet Disabled individuals are still massively underrepresented in retail and on

the runway. A 2022 report found that only 0.02% of fashion ad campaigns featured Disabled models, highlighting the urgent need for change (Walder, 2023). We can't leave it only to adaptive fashion brands – this must be covered by every designer, every brand, so that we have access to choice like our non-Disabled counterparts.

Disability representation in fashion is not just about visibility; it's about dignity, inclusion, and access. When Disabled people see themselves reflected in advertising, on the runway, and in retail spaces, it challenges outdated narratives and helps shift societal perceptions. It also ensures that the industry creates clothing that is functional and stylish for all bodies. Too often, Disabled people are forced to compromise on fashion because traditional designs fail to consider their needs. Everyone deserves to feel confident in what they wear.

Representation in fashion is more than just a trend; it is a movement toward true inclusivity that needs to be embedded behind and in front of the camera, from head office to shop floor. By hiring Disabled models, consulting with Disabled designers, and ensuring that adaptive clothing is available in mainstream retail, the fashion industry can take real steps towards accessibility. Disability is not a niche market; it is a reality for millions and that's before we include age-related Disability and temporary Disability. Inclusive design supports us all. Fashion has the power to change perception; it's past time the industry showed up for this community. 🙲

– Victoria Jenkins, CEO and Founder of Unhidden

Also, look at sports! Mainstream coverage of adaptive sports isn't always consistent, or equitable. They also don't get anywhere near the same coverage as non-adaptive sports and while major adaptive sporting events like the Paralympics and the Special Olympics have helped create visibility and recognition for Disabled athletes, other adaptive sports and events have had limited exposure, growth, and awareness.

These events have created an almost hierarchical valuation of Disabilities, where some categories of Disability receive more attention and resources than others. Athletes with less visible or more severe Disabilities might not get the same recognition, opportunities, or support, as evidenced by the separation of the Paralympics and the Special Olympics, with the latter often receiving less media attention and resources (Titone, 2024).

How the social and medical models impact representation

Now here we must have a conversation about the difference between representation and positive accurate representation because, goodness, do they mean very different things and can have very different desired consequences.

Imagine you're watching the blockbuster Hollywood movie of the year; it's about sailors sailing the high seas on their journey back to their island with the newly acquired treasures. On their journey, they encounter the villain, a one-legged evil pirate with broken speech and a scar across his face. The heroic sailors must fight to take down this evil pirate and escape to safety, which of course they do. Now, is this Disabled representation?

Wrong answer: yes, we have a Disabled character. Right answer:

although Disability is featured this is not an accurate or positive representation and therefore does not tick our boxes of representation.

Hello again, social model vs medical model of Disability, which we discussed in an earlier chapter. This is a pure and active demonstration of how we need to shift from the medical to the social model.

The medical model of Disability places first focus on the Disability, and the effect that a Disability has on an individual's inability to participate and engage fully within society, whereas the social model of Disability dictates that derogatory, offensive, or unpleasant language or terms should be identified in relation to Disabled people.

The social model also recognises the talents, aspirations, intelligence, and skills of Disabled people and does not adhere to the archaic stereotypes of the medical model.

Are we saying that Disabled characters can never be the baddies? Absolutely not, but if we are only ever the baddies and never the goodies, or never have a storyline which is an accurate portrayal of Disability, or we're only ever featured as cameos to tick a diversity box, or our Disabled characters are actually played by non-Disabled actors, then something has to change.

Positive Disabled representation is empowerment; it sets standards and showcases awareness, and is a catalyst for change, so it must therefore be done correctly. Because Disabled representation has historically been so poor, when we are portrayed as limited and stereotyped, this further perpetuates the very narratives that we are trying to destroy.

What does 'accurate' representations mean?

In the US, 95% of Disabled characters are played by non-Disabled people (Woodburn & Kopić, 2016). So even when we have Disability represented, our currently limited opportunities are being limited further based on the incorrect presumptions about the value and skills of the Disabled community. This is known as 'cripping up' – reinforcing the notion that Disability can be simulated or imitated over authentic lived experiences. This behaviour is deeply offensive to the Disabled community. This is not, and never will be, accurate and positive Disabled representation!

So, what do we mean by accurate representation? We mean representation that is diverse and reflective of lived experience. And when we say diverse, we mean that every type of Disability is represented, remembering that no two Disabled people are the same. This is not inspiration porn, or tokens, or always-struggling heroes – such narrow-minded and one-dimensional portrayals further demonise Disabled people and build walls of ableism, but are not recognised by the non-Disabled community. There is a difference. Autonomy, diverse experiences, agency, and talent – now that is Disabled representation.

Oh, and one more thing to add, we make up 17% of the world's population, and accurate representation means we should have our equal share of seats at the table, obviously.

Positive and accurate Disabled representation means just that, the clues are in the words! Representation should be a reflection of the size of the Disabled community, and reflect the positivity of it. Harmful inclusion is not the same as representation – the depiction of Disability must not only be more frequent but also more standardised in its positivity.

Globally, we do not have a unified understanding of Disability and this creates these disparities in society's acceptance and understanding and allows ableist narratives to run wild.

Unlearning ableist societal and cultural narratives about Disability

We witness the shock when a person learns that who they thought was our carer is actually our partner, or that a Disabled person is ordering rounds of shots for everyone at the bar. Non-Disabled people struggle to see Disabled people as contributing members or society who have needs and desires just like everyone else, and so ableism leads to narratives being created about Disabled people. Let's unpack some of the societal narratives about Disability.

The narrative: Disability is a tragedy

Disabled people's lives are so tragic. They have no friends, they can't work, it must be so hard for them.

People look at and treat Disability as if it's a personal tragedy, as if every Disabled person should come with their own tiny violin. This narrative stems from believing that all Disabled people are suffering and helpless, that we are mere objects to pity.

THE REALITY

We don't need your pity. Keep it. Yes, show empathy, as you should with every other single person, but don't expect us to whack out that tiny violin and play some Adele every time we share that we're Disabled. We don't need you to make us feel better or tell us that things can get better; we just need you to see us as a person, treat us as a person, and be open to us sharing our access needs. We don't need your pity, no thank you.

The narrative: The burden

Disabled people drain a country's resources; they're a drain on society, and too much money is spent on them. Why do we have to accommodate them when we're the majority?

Across society there are many people who consider Disabled people to be a drain on societal resources, including benefit and welfare systems. They view Disabled people as societal pariahs. Disabled people are asking or demand too much.

THE REALITY

Disabled people are not your burden. We pay taxes, we contribute to society, and you yourself benefit from universal design. Disabled people are contributing to art and culture. We created our own cultures. We are you one day. So, no, we aren't a burden on society; we navigate a society that places the burden of responsibility on us to educate others about these kinds of ableist narratives. We aren't a burden; we are contributors to society.

The narrative: Eternal innocence of a child

Disabled people are like children; they don't understand, they're so pure and innocent.

Some non-Disabled people treat Disabled people as children, regardless of their age, changing how they speak to them, how they treat them, and going as far as to talk about them to the 'grown-up' with them. Again, this happens no matter the Disabled person's age.

THE REALITY

We do not need you to treat us like children. We don't need you to speak to us like one either. And we for sure don't need you talking to the person with us as though they are our parent or guardian. If we need you to slow down or speak to us in a different style, let us communicate that to you, like the adults we are.

The narrative: The saintly Disabled person

Disabled people don't drink or take drugs, right? How could they? How would their poor bodies cope!

Society assumes that Disabled people make pure lifestyle choices because someone is bound to be making those choices for them.

THE REALITY

Disabled people, like everyone else, can have their habits; some of us bite our nails, some of us stuff ourselves with sweets, some enjoy a glass of wine, and some of us binge drink or abuse substances as a way to numb or self-medicate. Being Disabled does not make us exempt from the rollercoaster ups and downs of life, it doesn't cushion us from making good, bad, healthy, or unhealthy lifestyle choices. There is no one way to be Disabled.

The narrative: Sexless being

Disabled people are celibate. They don't have sex; how could they even do it?

People don't see Disabled people as desirable, leading them to believe that Disabled people themselves must not have desires. Disabled people aren't seen as sexy so why would they need or want sexy time with someone else?

THE REALITY

Newsflash: Disabled people have sex. We have good sex. We have bad sex. We have single partners, we have multiple partners. We have sex. Just like non-Disabled people get intimate, we too get intimate. We too have one-night stands, those awkward walks of shames the next day. We also flirt, date, fall in love, and have babies! Yes, we reproduce!

The narrative: Superhero and superhuman

Disabled people are superheroes or superhuman. Their Disabilities are what make them extraordinary, different, amazingly fantastical. Or on the flip side, in order to be seen or valued, Disabled people are made to feel that they need to be extraordinary and have exceptional talents.

THE REALITY

This narrative only puts pressure on Disabled people to perform or excel in order to be accepted. It's also infuriating for many Disabled people. It's okay for Disabled people to live normal lives, to go to work, to travel, to be a regular person. We don't need you to tell full grown adults that their Disability makes them a superhero. Now, it is important to note that for young Disabled people calling their Disabilities superhuman might seem like a great way to empower them, but there comes a point when we grow up and it moves from empowering to patronising.

The narrative: It's all in their head

People mistakenly believe that Disability is only a physical thing, ignoring non-visible conditions and the diversity of Disability. As well as this, Disabled people are often told that 'Disability is just in your head', 'You are more than your Disability, it is about your ability', 'Your Disability does not define you'.

THE REALITY

We won't go into a whole rant again about the diversity of Disability, but what we will say here is that while Disability is one piece of our identity, it is not a case of mind over matter, it is not in our head; it is an integral piece of our identity.

A lot of these narratives are formed because we aren't exposed to accurate representation of Disability, and this has had an impact on the social inclusion of Disabled people across society.

As you are learning, ableism is woven into every piece of our society, found within each industry, and while we've written chapters and chapters about all the ways this is ingrained, rather than recap them all below, we've focused on three key areas to paint a picture of how society has excluded us and now has the audacity to act surprised when we demand our rightful space.

Media

Inaccurate and harmful media portrayals of Disability have helped create harmful narratives and false perceptions of what it means to be Disabled. While we are seeing increased representation of Disability on the big screen, we need to remember that it is one Disabled person on screen, not the entirety of Disability being represented. We also have to remember when it comes to newspapers and media that we shouldn't always believe what we see or read.

Media portrayals of Disability often dismiss the complexity of Disability and limit social understanding of Disabled individuals. For example:

- Media campaigns that focus on suffering rather than empowerment.
- Narratives that position non-Disabled people as saviours.
- That one token Disabled character on screen, usually a person with visible Disability.
- The stereotyped portrayal of what it means to be Disabled.
- Inaccurate and false media campaigns targeting or dismissing Disability.

- Clickbait ableist headlines.
- Using facial disfigurement or visible Disabilities to portray villains or characters who are evil.

A survey conducted by Ipsos on behalf of the Business Disability Forum found that only 23% of Disabled respondents felt that images shared of Disability reflected their own experiences (Business Disability Forum, 2024). Now we know that when Disability is portrayed, it's not going to be everyone's experience, but we do at least expect some kind of reality, not some ableist stereotype – not some pity party or inspo porn.

These portrayals often serve to evoke sympathy or inspire others, rather than show Disabled people as complex, multifaceted individuals. The Inevitable Foundation found that 66% of audiences are unsatisfied with the current representations of Disability and mental health in film and TV; 25% of audiences also consider more than 90% of the depictions of Disability seen in the past year to be inauthentic (Inevitable Foundation, 2024).

Disabled people deserve better representation and more visibility in the media. For that young Disabled child sitting at home thinking they can't, for that young Disabled aspiring model or athlete who thinks they don't have a chance, and for all those with aspirations and hopes, seeing yourself represented is a powerful beacon and reminder of possibilities.

Sick influencers

We cannot write about the media without addressing what the western media has recently described as 'sick influencers'. As platforms like TikTok and Instagram have opened the world up to connecting and sharing lived experiences, we have seen witch hunts against Disabled and neurodivergent people who share their stories online. The western media has, in some areas, named and tried to shame these individuals.

When papers are putting targets on Disabled people's backs for daring to speak up in an ableist society, then those media and associated presses should be held accountable. It is never okay to attack, name, or shame Disabled people trying to support and help other Disabled people. After all, we know all too well how damaging the press is when it comes to creating harmful rhetoric and narratives about Disability and neurodiversity.

66 Authenticity is my vibe. I show up as my unfiltered, messy, neurodivergent, human self. I'm a Disabled 'influencer' (puke! But I believe everyone should be influential in their niche). I've shared the highs and the crippling lows, the business wins and the burnout. I share the reality of living with invisible Disabilities while running a business, raising a family, and helping others do the same. I also help people improve their money situation because navigating money as a neurodivergent person is HARD. So when a friend called and said, 'Maddy, they're talking about you on LBC', I was straight on the phone to give them what for! Being labelled a 'sickfluencer' in the national press wasn't just an attack on me, it was an attack on every person who has ever been told to hide their struggles for fear of being dismissed, judged, or ridiculed. The media suggested that talking about illness or Disability was manipulative. That sharing life with ADHD made me an attention seeker using Disability for personal gain. In reality, I talk about hidden Disabilities to break stigma and help people live better lives, including claiming benefits they are entitled to. We shouldn't be silenced. We shouldn't be ashamed

of our struggles and successes. If one person sees my TikTok and understands their brain or body better, I've done my job. Being Disabled isn't shameful. Claiming benefits doesn't make you a criminal. The more we own our soundtrack, the more people will realise ADHD isn't 'trendy'; it's a Disability. 99

– Maddy Alexandra-Grout, multi-award-winning entrepreneur, 'I'm not a "sickfluencer"; I'm a Disability champion'

Unlearning ableism in media

Unlearning ableism in the media starts with actually listening to Disabled people, representing the diversity of Disability, our different experiences, showing us as contributing members of society, who work, who shop, who are parents, and so on.

We need media outlets such as newspapers and blogs to be mindful of ableist language and to stop relying on and using outdated narratives or clickbait headlines to talk about or explore Disability-related topics. They need to stop running ableist, inaccurate stories that only aim to create smear campaigns. We only have to look at the media and what they have said about ADHD diagnosis – apparently it's over-diagnosed or it's a social trend – completely forgetting that more people are getting access to diagnosis, and due to better understanding of neurological thinking it has been recognised that it's not just boys who are ADHD.

Representation as a whole

Back to understanding representation as a whole, positive Disabled representation also plays a crucial role in promoting inclusion, equity, and diversity in our society. When Disabled people are not represented, we are effectively erased from conversation, marginalised, forgotten, pushed to the side. If you don't have Disabled people in the conversation, the outcome of that conversation is not going to be inclusive towards Disabled people, is it? Again, we say: nothing about us without us.

Strip it back for a second and imagine you have a group of people who are charged with creating a set of rules that decide what everybody needs, how they get it, and what tasks need to be done. This group of people create their rules and give them to another larger group of people who now have to go and complete them. If none of that original decision-making group share the same experiences, talents, or ways of living as the second larger group, the rules they create just won't work. Obvious, right? Well, that is exactly what is happening right now. Just look at the Disabled representation in our businesses, politics, and communities.

Ableism and discrimination are entrenched absolutely everywhere because we are not represented at the point of design in conversation. We are isolated and alienated, and this lack of representation is further perpetuating the notion that Disability should be hidden and under-valued, and it somehow makes us lesser, not worthy. By improving positive Disabled representation, we can pull down ableism barriers left, right, and centre, as we get it right from the beginning with accessibility, recruitment processes, inclusive fashion, and inclusive built environments.

Representation means that we can create a more inclusive and adapting society where the experiences of every person are identified, valued, and heard in building the foundations of our world. We have to eat at the same table, engage in the same games, and create a level playing field for opportunity and participation.

This word opportunity keeps cropping up, doesn't it? So, let's explore it

The equality of opportunity rhetoric stipulates that there is a transformation of opportunity and outcomes for Disabled people through the removal of ableism barriers and the promotion of inclusion. The equality of opportunity rhetoric stipulates that all individuals, whether they are Disabled or non-Disabled, are entitled to participate, contribute, and engage in the same manner as one another, through the creation and management of interacting opportunities that exist without barriers to Disabled people.

Equality of opportunity, in line with the premise of positive action and active intervention, stipulates the necessary and sustained removal of materials which do, or may, pose barriers to the participation, contribution, and engagement of Disabled people.

Equality of opportunity secures fair competition, to ensure that individuals are able to compete and participate at the same level without the existence of unfair advantage, unfair treatment, accessibility barriers, or discrimination. McTernan (2018) summarises the equality of opportunity rhetoric as 'equalising where people end up rather than where or how they begin'; regardless of Disability (beginning), an individual is entitled to the same political elective opportunities (ending), through the removal of equality of opportunity barriers such as implications, perceptions, and accessibility barriers. A Disabled person must be perceived as equal value, worth, talent, and ability as a person without a Disability. A Disabled person must be treated in the same non-discriminatory manner and receive fair treatment, process, and management as a person without a Disability.

So you see, we improve opportunity, we unlearn ableism, and we improve outcomes by creating better representation. For example, better representation in the design industry creates inclusive consumer choice, better political representation creates more inclusive legislation and policy, better representation in sports leadership creates more opportunity for participation. Representation holds a significant key to change and spans all areas of society.

We know that representation tears down attitudinal ableism and internalised ableism, and breaks down barriers across society but let's add something else to the mix: positive Disabled representation empowers, kicking internalised ableism's bum to the curb.

The research that we conducted at Disabled by Society showed that 95% of Disabled people had experienced ableism. We also found that only 1.5% of Disabled people had never experienced internalised ableism, and only 6.6% had never experienced mental health challenges as a direct result of their Disability (Disabled by Society, 2024).

Is inadequate Disabled representation the sole contributor to internalised ableism? No, but it is a massive factor that, if addressed, would have significant beneficial consequences. If we aren't seeing ourselves represented, if we can't even climb onto the ladders that move us up to being a representative ourselves, if we feel we aren't valued or portrayed, if we feel we aren't worthy of being shown, there is no wonder we feel the way we do. If we don't see ourselves represented, this perpetuates the notion that we are different and deserve to be separated off unseen. Disabled representation is key in smashing this state of play away.

How can we begin to improve Disabled representation?

So, now that we have learned why representation matters, we must now understand how to make it better. How can we each take responsibility to tear down this form of ableism and create more equity and opportunity for Disabled people through positive, inclusive, authentic, and diverse representation?

Accurate consultation

Disabled people need to be involved from beginning to end, and we must have an equal share of voice in the conversation (this does not just apply to representation). The voices of the Disabled community must be valued, respected, and heard, not as an afterthought or as a tick-box exercise – we have to be there too. Accurate consultation with those with lived experience creates positive, authentic, diverse, and inclusive processes for representation, shaping an accurate portrayal and action, when we think of the two meanings as both a noun and a verb that representation holds. If someone is to speak on our behalf, or portray our lived experience, or decide what we need or how we do things, it should come from a person who understands our experiences.

Diversifying the portrayal and imagery of Disability

We must diversify our portrayal and imagery of Disability. No two Disabled people are the same, nor are our experiences, our backgrounds, our feelings, our identities. We must make sure that in the representation of Disability, we are diverse. One Disabled person does not represent the whole Disabled community. Disabled representation does not mean one token voice or presence; it means having an accurate reflection of the 17% of the global population who identify as Disabled. One Disabled film cameo is not Disabled representation, a handful of Disabled MPs is not Disabled representation, one Disabled model on the catwalk is not Disabled representation. We can do so much better than this.

Representation means an accurate reflection of our society. We must prioritise showcasing and having a diverse community of people, with diverse experiences, diverse talents, diverse personalities, diverse Disabilities, and diverse identities – this is accurate representation. In tandem with this, we must challenge the imagery of Disability, the language we use, and the stories we portray. If you type the word Disability into a search engine and head to the news section, what will you find? Two things dominate: inspiration porn and negative stereotypes. We are either inspirational because of our achievements 'in spite of our Disabilities' or social scroungers, system abusers, lazy and unable to contribute to society. Where is the positive representation of Disability? Instances of this are few and far between, with outdated language and harmful stereotypes being the norm in conversation around Disability. We have already discussed how damaging this narrative is, so let's bloody change it.

Being open to feedback

We must open ourselves up to feedback, listen to criticism, be educated and learn, and be aware. Our research showed that 99% of Disabled people believe that non-Disabled people need more training and education on ableism (Disabled by Society, 2024). The responsibility to eradicate ableism through the improvement of Disabled representation and breaking down of barriers is on everybody. Disabled people unanimously agreed that everybody has to take accountability and responsibility for their actions and behaviours and that everybody should have access to safe, honest, and effective training and education.

There is no one lived experience, no one appearance, no one way to be Disabled, and no two individuals with the same condition or neurological conditions. Disability can impact anyone. Disability is part of the human experience. Society disables Disabled people and so does the ableism of others.

Our survey showed that 99% of Disabled people agree that it is for all of us to do and be better. And how do we be better? We learn from the very people who have lived experience, who have felt the consequences, who have the creativity to drive forward change (Disabled by Society, 2024). Feedback and education are critical – for too long our voices have been ignored and under-valued. Accurate and positive representation is a necessity, not a desire, and change comes through collaboration, active engagement, and openness.

Everybody has a role to play in improving representation, but it starts from the top down

Tying into the importance of feedback and education is recognising that change starts from the top down. We have to lead by example, diversify our teams across all levels, and ensure that Disabled people are present in conversations and consultations at all levels. Every person has a role to play in improving positive representation, from those in front and those behind the centre stage. From designers to manufacturers, to consultants to politicians, to healthcare workers to social leaders, everybody has a role to play. Through active commitment to diversification, we can create inclusivity, accessibility, and authenticity for more equitable and accurate Disabled representation. We should not be defining ourselves and living by the narrative that someone else has set.

The importance of identification

We must be critical in our thinking, seek to identify areas for improvement, and be proactive in seeking out ableism. If we sit back and allow ableism to pass us by, change moves ever further away into the distance. Change comes when we work towards it; change does not happen on its own. Adopt the mantra of positive action. Critically identify barriers and provide solutions, identify current and previous errors and provide solutions, highlight these errors and barriers to spread awareness and education, and foster an environment of critical discussion and representative input.

This end-to-end process of identification is not just about businesses or organisations; it is also about us as individuals, in what we engage in, the language we use, how we react, and how we interact. We must be alert and attentive, encouraging a critical active nature in ourselves, encouraging advocacy and self-advocacy to move towards better Disabled representation.

Representing Disability is needed in every area of our society: in healthcare, education, business, media, and so on. Representation means that Disabled people have a voice at the table; it means young and grown adults have people to look up to, to respect, to show them that we can do it, we can succeed, and we can thrive.

In conclusion

Let's conclude the conversation about Disabled representation and the role it has to play in moving forward in unlearning ableism. Where we are now is a place of under-valuing, underrepresenting, and incorrectly representing Disabled people, which is perpetuating the cycle of ableism through inaccessibility, lack of opportunities, and lack of participation.

Where do we need to be? We need to be in a place where as Disabled people we don't jump for joy when there is a Disabled person on TV because it is so unexpected, or cheer when a Disabled MP is elected, or all flock to the one shop that sells accessible clothing because we have nowhere else to go. We should have choice, we should have an opportunity, we should have the right to participate, and the right to be represented in the right way, without this negative narrative. It isn't just important, it is a necessity.

Representation promotes understanding, awareness, and equity for Disabled people, challenging stereotypes, promoting inclusion, embracing identity, and enhancing advocacy. We have to be active in our improvements; we have to be positive in our journey forward.

Remember those words we said right at the beginning of this chapter: conscious vs unconscious, accidental vs incidental, intentional vs unintentional. We have to move to a point where representation is happening unconsciously and unintentionally because it is just part of everyday life! But to get to that point we have to be intentional; representation does not improve by accident, we have to influence and narrate the story we want to tell, and we all have a responsibility to make accurate and positive representation a reality.

We should note the incredible work of individuals and organisations around the world who are challenging our current reality and forging a path ahead for better Disabled representation, showing that authentic positive action creates inclusive processes for all, educating and ending negative bias. We need everyone to join this action and we must all share responsibility and accountability. Change comes through allyship and proactivity. Everybody deserves to be represented and feel confident in their future.

For the final time in this chapter we say: nothing about us without us.

CHAPTER 11

Unlearning Ableism:
Education

> **Disabled people spend their lives in the role of 'educator', which is ironic considering the education system itself has, and continues to create, many barriers for Disabled people.**

Access to education is recognised around the world as a fundamental human right, a right which for many Disabled people is not met.

The Universal Declaration of Human Rights, which was adopted in 1948, states that 'everyone has the right to education'. Since then, a number of other international treaties, as well as domestic laws, have been adopted to reaffirm this statement including the UNESCO Convention against Discrimination in Education (1960), the International Covenant on Economic Social and Cultural Rights (1966), and the Convention on the Rights of Persons with Disabilities (2006).

Under these laws and universal acknowledgement of the importance of education you might assume that access to education for Disabled people would be equitable, but that would be wrong. Ableism in education is rife, with devastating consequences for individuals and their parents/caregivers, who in many instances are a Disabled person's first advocate.

But this conversation about education isn't just about the receipt of education for Disabled people. It's also about the importance of education around Disability and ableism for non-Disabled people.

Did you know that 96.8% of Disabled people do not believe enough is being done to address ableism within our society (Disabled by Society, 2024)?

So, if everyone is in agreement that not having access to adequate and equitable education is one of the biggest barriers then why are Disabled people consistently denied fair and equitable treatment in schools, colleges, and universities? And additionally, if there are so many international treaties about fairness between differences of identity, why are we consistently failing to educate on inclusion, equity, accessibility, and Disability awareness?

To answer this, we must first understand why access to education is so important, and provide context to everything we are going to be discussing.

- **Empowerment:** Education is empowerment. Through the provision of knowledge, skills, confidence, and assets we are able to make more informed decisions, take more control of our life paths, and, above all, have openness to choice.

- **Opportunity:** Education is often the key to unlocking economic opportunities and improving circumstances. Those with better access to education have more openness to job choice, higher salaries and earning potentials (if for a moment we pretended that Disability barriers were not something else to contend with).

- **Social mobility:** Education is a fundamental key in opening systemic cycles of changing circumstances, providing people with the opportunity to move along and up social and economic ladders. Education allows for attainment.

- **Personal development:** Education helps people develop critical and diverse skills, creativity, and aspiration for learning, enhancing our personal growth and awareness.

- **Social connection:** Education provides an environment to connect with peers, learn from others, and begin to understand the complexities of relationships.

- **Global competitiveness:** In today's ever-increasingly interconnected and competitive world, access to quality education is essential for individuals and allowing them to compete effectively on a level playing field. Education is individual and societal empowerment, access to opportunities, social mobility, access to choice, and access to competition.

It's key to remember that throughout everything we are about to discuss in relation to education, there is a phrase we are going to use time and time again: early intervention!

Early intervention

This means identifying and providing effective, accessible, and positive support to children and young Disabled people who are at a higher risk of negative outcomes. It means being proactive, not reactive, preventing problems before they arise or tackling them immediately and head-on when they do, before they get worse. Early intervention reduces risk factors, and increases factors in a person's life which act in a protective manner.

Early intervention typically targets four key areas: physical, cognitive, behavioural, and social and emotional development – promoting skills which will have the biggest benefit for an individual to take through life.

To be clear, this does not mean eradicating features of Disability, teaching a child how to 'hide' their condition, or forcing a Disabled person not to use their mobility aid. Early intervention is about the development of personal skills, independence, and enhancing of natural attributes, equipping us with the necessary skills needed later in life. Effective early intervention enhances these skills and promotes development tailored to an individual.

If early interventions are not imposed, Disabled people do not get access to education that is accessible and equitable, and environments that go beyond a one-size, non-Disabled, neurotypical majority.

Early intervention and access to education is so important because children and those who have experienced a significant life change, such as the acquisition of a Disability, are statistically proven to learn better than others. This is due to several reasons (but remember that Disability is incredibly diverse and no two people's experiences or ways of learning are the same):

- **Neuroplasticity:** Our brains during these times are much more malleable and adaptable than others. We are more easily able to learn new information and skills, as our brains are developing and forming new neural connections. While neuroplasticity is present throughout life, it is especially pronounced in early childhood, making early educational interventions particularly effective. This is supported by research on brain development (Cunnington, 2019).

- **Curiosity:** When we are young, we are naturally curious about learning, experiences, and discovery. As children and when we find ourselves in a different circumstance, we have a lack of perceived notions (and this is a big one we will come back to later) and are often more open-minded. We don't have the same level of fear of failure and judgement as others, having not yet absorbed and activated internalised ableism.

- **Learning experience:** We have the opportunity to play, explore, and engage in alternative ways, finding what works for each of us and developing our methods. As we develop, so do our retention and skills. Children have a growth mindset; our skills and talents are developed through perseverance and nurture, as we are allowed space to make mistakes, take risks, and foster personal attitudes.

So, with all of that being said, it is quite clear that if we fail to provide Disabled people with accessible and effective access to education, we are only further entrenching ableism in our society as we fail to equip them with the same opportunities to reap the benefits of education.

It should be no surprise to learn that in a survey by the National Autistic Society (2024), almost 74% of parents and carers said their child's needs were not met in school, and nearly a third of parents (30%) had had to use the legal system to get their children the right provision.

In developing countries approximately 90% of Disabled children do not receive structured education (World Health Organization, 2011).

Research shows that Disabled students frequently experience lower academic success and retention rates compared to their non-Disabled peers (Claricoats, 2024).

The Office for National Statistics (2019) reported that Disabled people were less likely to have a degree-level qualification, with 21.8% of Disabled people having any degree compared with 38.0% of non-Disabled people. The proportion of Disabled people who had no qualifications was more than two and a half times that of non-Disabled people (16.1% compared with 6%).

A survey conducted by the Department for Education (2020a) revealed that 22% of teachers felt unprepared to meet the needs of pupils with special educational needs (SEN).

Ofsted Parent View data revealed that nearly a third (29%) of parents of pupils with special educational needs would not recommend their child's secondary school to other parents (Centre for Social Justice, 2021).

And a 2018/19 survey found that only 14.9% of parents of Disabled children surveyed said their child's school provided information in an accessible format without them needing to make additional requests (Mencap, n.d.).

This data from the UK paints a grim picture. It evidences a massive failure to provide Disabled people with equitable opportunities to learn, feel empowered, and develop.

Access to education for Disabled people, even when the education provided is meant to have been designed for Disabled people, is still riddled with inaccessibilities and ableism. Inaccessible built environments such as classrooms and play facilities that students are not able to use or navigate, skills training which focuses solely on neurotypical development and encouragement, failure to provide adjustments and additional support, failure to provide sensory strategies and equipment, belittling language and behaviour towards individuals or groups…we could write a whole chapter just giving you examples!

66 I'm Avril, an intersectional non-white Disabled female born to parents from Asia and Africa. I got epilepsy in childhood. Anti-seizure medication slowed my mentation significantly.

I sat my first exam isolated aged 11. Despite school records, subsequent exams were sans extra time, thus I only completed lengthy art exams. A teacher tried to exclude me from a significant field trip due to epilepsy despite GP, consultant neurologist, and parental support.

After my first degree, I began a post-graduate certificate in education. I immediately told pupils about my epilepsy, with the school's agreement. I had 16 classes, and a form group whose various regular teachers shadowed me. I had a seizure, and a pupil noticed and helped me. My supervising tutor in school bullied me and on return from a school trip, I found that my supervising tutor had engineered a way to oust me two and a half months short of qualifying. I felt it was because of my earlier seizure.

In my student teaching experience, mandatory GP appointments downgraded anyone with asthma, dyslexia, or epilepsy to a C grade, reducing teaching opportunities on qualification. Extra exam time was not given annually, despite schools knowing medical needs. I also experienced bullying, discrimination, stigmatisation, and stereotype tropes from teachers.

I would advise anyone in a similar position to plan ahead for coursework with deadlines, to read over the summer, and to formally request adequate extra time for exams annually. Schools need to educate young people about Disability to break down barriers. Disabled student teachers should not be marked down in their grades, and schools must accept bullied Disabled student teachers' lived experiences and deal with ableist bullies. Ableist trauma can be removed by education, inclusion, understanding needs, and removing barriers. Equitable and accessible opportunities for Disabled people must be created. "

– Miss Avril Coelho

Every Disabled child's experience of the education system is different, and for millions around the world this means attending 'specialist education', specifically providing for Disabled children with diverse needs. Now we do have to say that we personally do not agree with the term special education, but to avoid confusing things, we will use this for now.

'Specialist education' facilitates specialist trained staff, adapted curriculums, specialist facilities, and staff who often work closely with other professional services such as care providers, healthcare, and therapists. This type of education is designed to provide tailored education and support to children who have specific learning, emotional, or physical needs that mean they are not able to be in mainstream education. As we said, every child's experience is different, and it is important to recognise the lifeline that these schools provide for children, their families and carers, creating a safe space that benefits physical and mental well-being, as well as providing respite.

- SEN schools are equipped to provide individualised learning plans, addressing the unique strengths and areas of development for each child. This allows students to progress at their own pace without the pressure of competing with peers who may have different needs.

- With fewer students in each class, children receive more focused attention from teachers, allowing for a more supportive and interactive learning experience. This can be particularly helpful for children who may find it more difficult in larger, more chaotic classrooms.

- SEN schools have teachers, therapists, and support staff who are trained to work with students with specific needs. This expertise ensures that students are given the right support and their educational experiences are structured to encourage individual skills and talents.

- These schools often provide a more nurturing and understanding environment, where children feel less stigmatised for their Disability. It can be a space where they feel accepted, understood, and encouraged to express themselves freely, reducing anxiety or the feeling of being judged.

- Many SEN schools are equipped with resources, technology, and physical spaces designed to accommodate different needs. This includes things like sensory rooms, mobility aids, and specific learning tools that make education more accessible.

- SEN schools often prioritise social, emotional, and life skills development. They help students build self-esteem, confidence, and unique skills critical for their future well-being and independence.

- Mainstream schools can sometimes create stress or anxiety

for children who find the environment overwhelming. SEN schools often have access to a range of support services like speech therapy, occupational therapy, and behavioural therapy, integrated into the daily routine. This holistic approach helps address any non-academic barriers a child might face.

We cannot discuss SEN without highlighting that for many Disabled people the term SEN carries a stigma, trauma, and feelings from past ableist experiences. To be a child labelled with special education needs was in many cases to be treated differently. It meant special classes, away from the other children. It meant segregation. It meant a different way of being educated. There is a lot of debate on whether the term special needs is ableist and we do believe it to be so. While the term is recognisable within education, we also have to remember that Disabled people have historically not had the power or voice within these spaces; therefore the term special needs is a way for non-Disabled people to distinguish the difference between what is perceived as 'normal needs' and what is 'special'. Disabled people can have access needs – human needs – that don't make us special. This kind of language is not empowering and it carries a stigma.

We also have to recognise the difficulties and barriers experienced by parents and caregivers of Disabled children in education. It is no easy task to get your Disabled child the support they require – the adjustments and accommodations they need, the empathy and understanding they need. Trying to have a child placed in accessible education or to be even supported in mainstream education is an extremely exhausting, challenging, and thankless task.

In many cases, parents of Disabled children have spent years fighting for their child's right to an equitable education, making endless trips back and forth from the school to speak to the teacher, the principal, the occupational therapists, or whoever is going to listen. There are sleepless nights, a fear for your child's future, and having to repeat the same conversations over and over again until someone listens.

Parents, guardians, and carers, we salute you. You are our first advocates, you are the voice of our inclusion and we know it is not and was not easy. But we want you to know we grow into adults who have the utmost love and respect for your tireless, thankless task of trying to ensure that your child has an education. We know there is not enough support, there are not enough resources. We know that ableism prevents you from accessing support for your child.

There is a massive misconception when discussing Disabled people's education that all Disabled children attend specialist education. This is wildly incorrect.

In the UK, less than 10% of children with SEN attend specialist schools. Specifically, in England, 9.3% of pupils with SEN were enrolled in special schools during the 2019/20 academic year. Similar trends are seen in Northern Ireland (9.8%) and Wales (5.3%) for that same period. The vast majority of children with SEN in the UK are educated within mainstream schools, with specialist provisions being available to only a small portion of the population (Department for Education, 2020b). Similarly, in the US, approximately 7.5% of students with Disabilities attend separate special schools, according to the US Department of Education's National Center for Education Statistics (2020).

Most children access education through mainstream schools, and with this comes a whole host of ableism on our plates too. You're probably thinking, 'But we didn't have anyone in our class who was Disabled!' Remember that Disability is incredibly diverse and intersectional; it does not just mean physical, visible conditions. Disability can be non-physical and non-visible, so you can't always 'know' just by looking at somebody!

Ableism within our education systems is not just in our specialist schools. You'll be unsurprised to learn that it is spread throughout the education system in mainstream education as well (understatement of the century). Want some examples? Over a third of SEN children (36%) said they often, always, or 'some of the time' felt lonely, compared to 23% of other children. Only 14.1% of Disabled people said they were taught about ableism, and therefore their rights and protections, in education, and of those who sought education about ableism, 62.4% said they had to teach themselves (Disabled by Society, 2024).

And what does ableism look like in mainstream education? Again, we come in with a potentially endless list:

- Inaccessible classrooms and facilities.
- Barriers to participation.
- Failure of personalised care plans.
- Inflexible structures and requirements.
- Purely academic achievement-based rewards systems.
- Neurotypical learning frameworks.
- A lack of early intervention.
- A lack of Disability support.

If you ask any person who went through education as a Disabled person whether they faced any barriers because of their Disability, their answer will always be yes. Shall we circle back to what we said at the very beginning, to the universal human rights declaration, 'everyone has the right to education', education that is fair and equal – do we think this is happening?

Education is unanimously identified by the Disabled community as one of the largest problems in our society in carrying systemic ableism. And the consequences? Remember what we discussed in why education is so important – opening opportunities, social mobility, skills and enhancement of talents, development, participation, and choice? To fail to provide education free from ableism is further entrenching the discrimination and ostracisation of Disabled people throughout society, and entrenching internalised ableism because from a young age we adopt the values that we perceive the world to have of us – that we aren't even worthy of receiving basic human rights as children.

'School days are the best days of your life'

66 That's what we're told. And for many non-Disabled people, that might be true. But for a lot of Disabled people, school is the first place they realise they're different – and the first place they experience discrimination.

Being made to stand at the front of the class to see a whiteboard. Missing lessons because the materials aren't accessible. Sitting through Christmas films with no audio description or subtitles. Being left out of playground games. Going on school trips where nothing can be touched. Being told you can't take part in certain subjects because you're a 'health and safety risk'.

None of this is exaggeration. These were my experiences as a blind child in the late 1990s and 2000s. And I went to a good, specialist school, designed for kids like me. What would I have faced in a mainstream school?

But it doesn't have to be like that.

School could be the place where Disabled young people learn that it's barriers – not their impairments – that disable them. It could be where they figure out what adjustments work for them and what they need for the workplace, when and how to ask for them. It could be where non-Disabled young people grow up understanding Disability as just a normal part of life – like having different hair colours.

Because when education is inclusive, Disabled young people don't just learn better; they grow up prepared to take on life as Disabled adults. And non-Disabled young people grow up knowing how to build a world where inclusion isn't an afterthought.

That's your job, as someone reading this chapter. You can make all of that possible if you want to, and now you're going to read how... 99

– Robbie Crow, Strategic Disability Lead at the BBC, and an advocate of the social model of Disability

Disabled people in education need better access and inclusion for a multitude of reasons, in addition to the cycle of internalised ableism. Education is at the forefront of equality and equity; it is a basic human right, and all people, whether Disabled or not, should have equal access to quality education. This provision promotes inclusion and accessibility throughout our society. Education plays a crucial role in our development and growth, enabling us to harness our skills and unique attributes to compete on a level playing field, access choice, and fulfill our potential. We gain the knowledge, skills, and confidence to make informed decisions, advocate for ourselves, and participate, promoting independence and self-determination.

Education is also a necessary tool for socialisation and interaction, fostering belonging, community, support, and connection to reduce the prevalence of isolation that most Disabled people face. Education equips and prepares us for the future, and should meet the needs of all people, regardless of adjustments or tailoring. Education is Thor's hammer against ableism.

So, what can we do?

Eradicating ableism, as we have discussed in every single chapter of this book, is everybody's responsibility, at every level. We all need to take accountability. Governing bodies must take accountability in the funding and provision of better resources; teachers must have better access to training, support, and awareness to identify and support students. We need to be proactive, take conscious positive action, break down cyclical systems, examine conscious biases, anticipatory duty, and so on – you've heard it before, and more on understanding these sentiments can be found in our final chapter.

And a big one, something you've heard time and time again throughout this book. There needs to be better understanding and awareness about Disability, equity, ableism, and accessibility throughout society, from the top to the bottom, left and right, here, there, and everywhere, which leads us very conveniently into our next discussion point.

When we talk of ableism in education, we aren't just talking about access to education for Disabled people; we are also talking about the desperate need for better education and awareness on Disability in our educational systems. In our survey (Disabled by Society), 87.9% of Disabled people said there needs to be more education and training in understanding ableism, and 93.8% of Disabled people believed there was not sufficient education about Disability and ableism in the education system. A giant key to dismantling ableism is staring us in the face and we've said it time and time again: education, education, education.

Where do we start?

- Integrate Disability awareness into the curriculum to educate all students about different Disabilities, intersectionality, and the barriers we face.

- Foster an environment where inclusion is a core value, encouraging students and staff to understand and be aware of Disability.

- Create flexible, individual, or tailored learning environments that accommodate different learning styles and Disabilities.

- Provide alternative, accessible methods of teaching and assessment, teaching universal design and usability from the beginning.

- Offer continued professional development to educators on inclusive teaching strategies, Disability awareness, and how to recognise and challenge ableism in the classroom.

- Ensure that teaching materials, books, and media include diverse representations of Disabled people in a positive and empowering light.

- Promote student-led initiatives and peer support groups that advocate for inclusivity, and challenge ableist attitudes and behaviours, while also providing a safe space for Disabled and neurodivergent people to come together.

- Ensure that physical spaces, learning materials, and technology are accessible to all students.

- Have clear, written policies that prohibit ableist behaviour, including bullying, discrimination, and exclusion, and provide mechanisms for reporting and addressing such issues.

- Facilitate group work, projects, and extracurricular activities that encourage collaboration between students with and without Disabilities, breaking down social barriers and systematic segregation.

- Engage families and communities in promoting inclusive attitudes and practices, and provide resources to help them understand and support students with Disabilities both in and outside school.

And in the long term?

- Strengthen and enforce laws and policies surrounding the inclusion of Disabled people in education. Our legal frameworks should ensure that schools are required to provide equal educational opportunities for all students, regardless of Disability. These laws need to explicitly state that inclusion isn't just about access, but about meaningful participation and appropriate support. Clear accountability measures must be in place to ensure that schools comply with inclusion mandates. This includes regular reviews of the implementation of inclusive practices and policies. Policies should promote equity, by not only ensuring access but also ensuring that Disabled students have equal opportunities for academic success, extracurricular activities, and social inclusion. Inclusive education is a fundamental human right, not a privilege, and there must always be an avenue for legal recourse for students who are discriminated against based on their Disabilities.

- Reduce segregation of Disabled students while maintaining tailored support. Inclusive classrooms should be the standard for all educational bodies, with strategies in place to reduce the unnecessary segregation of Disabled students, without compromising individual needs. For students who require more specialised support, collaborative models (such as co-teaching or differentiated instruction) should be encouraged. Mainstream education teachers, special education teachers, and support staff must work together to create an environment where the barriers for Disabled students are actively tackled, allowing all to thrive. Personalised accommodations and adjustments should be available, with appropriate resources provided to enable inclusion without sacrificing academic rigour. Tailored support can come in many forms, such as assistive technologies, therapy, and flexible teaching methods.

- Infuse accessibility into all buildings, from the point of design, and as a set standard for all educational authorities. Accessibility standards for school buildings should be a priority in both new constructions and renovations. These standards should go beyond wheelchair access to include sensory accommodations, such as quiet spaces for students with sensory processing differences, and soundproofing to minimise distractions. Schools should be designed with flexibility and individuality in mind, ensuring that classrooms can be easily adapted for different needs such as adjustable furniture, assistive technologies, and visual or tactile signage for students with sensory differences. Transportation to and from school should also be made accessible and available for Disabled students, ensuring that buses, school entrances, and other infrastructure accommodate a wide range of needs, from mobility challenges to sensory sensitivities. The creation of accessible environments also means that digital accessibility, including school websites, online learning platforms, and educational tools, must be incorporated from the outset, following Web Content Accessibility Guidelines standards to ensure that all students can access online content.

- Ensure that Disability awareness and education are a core component of teacher training. Teacher preparation programmes must include comprehensive training on Disability awareness. Educators should be taught from the outset how to recognise and support students. Training should not only focus on practical strategies for students but also on changing social attitudes towards Disability, ensuring that teachers understand the value of inclusive education and are equipped to challenge ableist beliefs and behaviours, contributing to the breaking down of systemic ableist attitudes. In addition to initial training, ongoing professional development on Disability issues should be mandatory throughout teachers' careers to keep them updated on best practices, legal changes, and new technologies.

- Ensure that educational bodies recognise and support early diagnosis. Schools should be proactive in recognising potential Disabilities and neurodivergence and providing early intervention, and ensuring that these are followed up with timely assessments. Schools should create collaborative processes with healthcare providers, parents, guardians, or carers and specialised professionals to support early diagnosis and intervention. This can include offering screenings for various conditions like dyslexia, ADHD, or speech delays, and helping families access the necessary services and support. Early intervention is crucial for ensuring that Disabled children receive the support they need before they fall behind academically or socially. Programmes like Response to Intervention or early literacy support can be implemented to ensure that students receive assistance as soon as barriers are identified.

We have to start changing the ableist patterns in our generations to come, to break the cycle of discrimination and ensure that we are fulfilling the basic human rights of everyone to be able to access equity in education and reap the benefits from it.

We have to unlearn the ableism in education if we are ever to empower future generations of Disabled people.

CHAPTER 12

Unlearning Ableism: Recruitment and Workplaces

> 'Oh, goody, another inaccessible application. Another ableist recruitment process. Will I even be able to request adjustments/ accommodations?' 'If this is how it is at the recruitment stage, how bad will it be if they hire me?' If we had a pound for every ableist recruitment process or workplace we have encountered, we wouldn't even need to work because we'd be rich.

The traumas of being a Disabled person seeking employment or being an employed Disabled person cannot be trivialised:

- Barrier-riddled recruitment processes.
- Exclusionary job descriptions.
- Untrained and unaware hiring teams.
- Ableist experiences when interacting with hiring teams.
- Rejected for self-identifying.
- Ghosted when making an adjustment or accommodation request.
- Discriminated against because you are Disabled.

These experiences don't just happen in isolation. This is what it means to be a Disabled person trying to find employment. It's one barrier after another, fresh new ableist experiences behind every application – behind every job offer, within every workplace, behind every unsupportive manager's misguided intent.

It shouldn't surprise you to learn that Disabled people are almost twice as likely to be unemployed than their non-Disabled peers (Scope, n.d.a). Disabled people navigate a job market not designed for them, a job market which favours non-Disabled people, causing Disabled people to bounce from one workplace to another, trying to find that all-singing, all-dancing inclusive employer.

We are searching for an employer where:

- we can be our authentic selves, Disability and all
- our access needs can be met
- managers are equipped and supportive of Disabled employees
- we are respected, valued, and supported
- we feel belonging
- we have opportunities
- we see ourselves represented.

Sadly, for us, trying to find an inclusive employer can feel a bit like the Hunger Games – the odds are never in our favour.

A study by the International Labour Organisation (2018) reported that there were an estimated 386 million working-age Disabled people globally, but yet up to 80% of these employable individuals were unable to find work due to various barriers, including discrimination or lack of adjustments and accommodations.

If you asked an employer about this, they would probably tell you that there is a lack of candidates. In fact, 47% of business leaders believe that the key barrier to the recruitment and retention of Disabled people is a lack of candidates (The Valuable 500, 2021). So, we have employers telling us there are no Disabled candidates, and Disabled people struggling to find employment – what is happening?

Well, to paint a better picture, it's worth highlighting the employment rate for Disabled people around some parts of the world.

- 53% of Disabled people in the UK are employed, compared to 82% of non-Disabled people (Scope, n.d.a).

- 19.1% of Disabled people in the US are employed, compared to 63.7% of non-Disabled people (US Bureau of Labor Statistics, 2021).

- 50.6% of Disabled people in Europe are employed, compared to 74.8% of non-Disabled people (European Parliament, 2020).

- 53.4% of Disabled people in Australia are employed, compared to 83.2% of non-Disabled people (Australian Bureau of Statistics, 2020).

- 65.1% of Disabled people in Canada are employed, compared to 80.1% of non-Disabled people (Statistics Canada, 2023).

- 36% of Disabled people in India are employed, meaning nearly 64% are unemployed (Sharma, 2021).

A survey conducted by global Disability job board, Evenbreak (2020), revealed that 82% of Disabled job seekers believed the main barrier to sourcing suitable employment was finding employers who were genuinely Disability friendly.

But yet organisations fail to gain and retain Disabled people. They fail to represent Disability; they fail to go beyond mere tokenistic words of inclusion. Leadership teams may claim, 'Disabled people don't apply for our roles' or, 'There are no Disabled people working here.' The reality is, of course, that Disabled people are already applying for roles and working within these organisations; it's just much more likely that these organisations are failing to provide an accessible recruitment process and failing to create anti-ableist inclusive workplace cultures. They are failing to create a sense of belonging for Disabled people and failing to create workplaces that retain us.

Performative Disability inclusion

'We are the most inclusive, accessible company.' 'We provide equal opportunities for everyone.' 'We are the most amazing diverse organisation.' We have all heard companies screaming and shouting from the rooftops about how inclusive they are, how they are the most amazing super-duper award-winning organisation, patting themselves on the back for telling us all how incredibly inclusive they are. So much so, that when you visit their website you will find pages bursting with words of inclusion and a trophy case proudly displaying awards and accreditations, proclaiming this organisation to be the most equitable, the most inclusive, the most equal organisation. The most 'insert title' here…

These awards and accreditations have become a way for organisations to promote and sell themselves as inclusive employers for all. But on closer inspection we often realise that the websites are actually inaccessible and lack any kind of Disability representation, and if we look further and explore the origins of some of these awards and accreditations, we find that the companies operating some of them have also some pretty questionable accessibility standards, while others are self-obtained and self-certified.

In the UK, the Disability Confident scheme, a government-run initiative aimed at helping employers to attract and retain Disabled people, and Disabled people to recognise inclusive employers, revealed that 37% of Disability Confident employers had not recruited at least one Disabled person since joining up to the scheme (Department for Work and Pensions, 2022). This begs the question, if you are sticking a logo or an award on your website like a proud peacock, surely you need to be doing the work? Surely you need to be taking action, not just talking the talk. Disabled people should have the confidence that the organisation they are applying to is going to be accessible and inclusive for them, that if they are successful they have the same opportunities to succeed. And that starts with the recruitment process.

Recruitment

In this section we will dissect how to create accessible, anti-ableist recruitment processes, helping organisations to attract and gain Disabled talent.

But please understand, the change you are going to be making in your recruitment process also needs to be happening internally. It is not an either/or. If you are creating a recruitment process that is accessible, but your culture is a cesspool of barriers, then you are going to set Disabled people up to fail and you will not retain us.

So, buckle up and let's unlearn the ableism in your recruitment processes.

Disability-confident recruiters

Hiring teams are not being taught about the ableism they are contributing to in the hiring process, whether it's in the job description they are crafting or the way they communicate with candidates. Scope (n.d.c) highlights that 37% of Disabled applicants believe employers will not hire them because of their impairment but despite this, Disabled people continue to apply for 60% more jobs than non-Disabled people.

Your hiring teams need to have training on accessibility, ableism, the diversity of Disability, bias, and adjustments and accommodations. They should know the process for making adjustments and accommodations, how to have conversations without ableist language, and how to follow through with an accessibility request. They should read this book.

Role requirements

Role requirements, we get it, they are an integral way of qualifying candidates for a position, but if you are not focusing on the essential requirements of the role, you risk excluding Disabled candidates. The essential requirements of a role are the core tasks and responsibilities that a person needs to be able to perform to succeed in the job. This means focusing on what exactly the person will be doing in the role, and what specific skills, knowledge, and abilities are needed to carry out those tasks.

Sticking to the essential skills of the role ensures that you are providing an equitable experience for everyone. Equity, as we know, is recognising an individual's circumstances. For a Disabled person reading a job description, equity is the last thing we feel when the language is ableist and the requirements unclear or excluding. Ableist job requirements are written in a way that tells us you only want one type of candidate, one kind of person, someone who is non-Disabled, someone without access needs.

We get it: some roles will automatically disqualify some candidates. Jamie isn't going to be applying to be a lollipop person, and Celia is not going to apply to be a food critic any time soon. So yes, there will be some role requirements where certain things are needed, but for others we need to change the narrative of, 'Well, this is how it's always been done'. It's time to learn to be flexible, to begin considering that there are alternative ways of doing things. Consider these alternatives:

- Rather than standing at a cashier, a person might need a chair.

- Rather than using a standard desk, a person might need a standing desk or an adjustable workstation.

- Rather than requiring verbal communication, a person might use a speech-to-text device or a sign language interpreter.

- Rather than lifting heavy boxes, a person might use assistive equipment like a trolley or hoist.

- Rather than attending in-person meetings, a person might require video conferencing options.

- Rather than writing by hand, a person might use voice recognition software or a keyboard.

- Rather than working a fixed schedule, a person might need flexible hours or remote working options.

- Rather than navigating a large office space, a person might need a workstation closer to amenities or an accessible entrance.

- Rather than using a mouse, a person might use keyboard shortcuts or adaptive technology.

- Rather than requiring face-to-face customer interaction, a person might provide support via email or chat.

Sound familiar? It should. These are workplace adjustments and accommodations, simple yet powerful tools or changes that remove barriers and challenge the idea that there is only one way of doing things. There *is* more than one way of doing things.

ADJUSTMENTS AND ACCOMMODATIONS

In most developed countries there are legal frameworks that require an employer to make reasonable adjustments and accommodations for Disabled employees. In the UK, it is the Equality Act 2010, in the US it's the Americans with Disabilities Act, in the European Union it's the EU Employment Equality Directive (2000). We personally do not like to use the word reasonable because it is too open to interpretation. The law of course dictates what is reasonable for an employer and what is not.

To us, reasonable implies that there is a threshold where adjustments and accommodations are reasonable, rather than how essential they are for a person in a role. What is unreasonable, of course, should be written and clearly outlined in an adjustments and accommodations policy. But when you start the conversation about adjustments and accommodations with the negative, 'reasonable', you are already waving red flags at us. Instead use 'workplace adjustments' or 'workplace tools', which says exactly what it means on the tin.

Employers tend to believe that workplace adjustments and accommodations are expensive. Yet in the US, nearly 50% of workplace adjustments and accommodations for Disabled individuals incur no cost to employers, and for those that do have a one-time cost, the median expenditure is $300 (Job Accommodation Network, 2024). In the UK NHS Employers reports that most workplace adjustments cost less than £100, while many cost nothing at all (NHS Employers, 2023). That's a free or small cost to improve the health and well-being of an employee, and of course not being liable for failing to comply with legal requirements. Adjustments and accommodations offer Disabled people the opportunity to navigate the workplace in a safe, accessible way, and to be able to perform in their role.

Now think back to those role requirements we discussed, and let's tackle some of the ableist requirements that adjustments and accommodation could have supported:

'MUST HAVE A DRIVING LICENCE'

If the role is a bus driver or a racing car driver, we get it, you need to drive. But if the role is office based, why is a licence required? This requirement rules out those of us who are Disabled and legally not permitted to drive. If the role does require some travel between locations, then other more accessible travel arrangements can be secured. Buses, trains, public transport, or private transport are viable adjustments and accommodations to make for a person who is unable to drive.

'MUST HAVE EXCELLENT VERBAL COMMUNICATION'

This requirement can potentially exclude Disabled people with speech impairments, d/Deaf, neurodivergence, and so on, making them question if they should or could apply. Could written communication be just as effective? Are there any adaptations to be considered, or are there technical adjustments and accommodations that could be used to support an individual?

'MUST BE ABLE TO WORK IN A FAST-PACED ENVIRONMENT'

This statement deters candidates who may take extra time to complete a task, and it is a one-size-fits-all approach to workplace culture. When you say fast-paced, do you mean a person has to move a lot, which may restrict some individuals with mobility needs without an adjustment or accommodation, or are you just trying to tell us you expect long hours, no breaks, and one team doing the job of three? Not only does this statement scream exclusion, but it also screams toxic workplace.

'MUST BE STRONG' OR 'MUST BE ABLE TO LIFT' OR 'MUST BE ABLE TO STAND FOR LONG PERIODS'

These kinds of requirements rely on being physically capable of doing things. Not everyone can stand for long periods of time – imagine a person with scoliosis, or someone using a wheelchair – so can you understand how this statement of standing would deter them? Relying on physicality will automatically disqualify many Disabled candidates. Think of it this way: hiring someone to work in a call centre and saying they must be able to stand for long periods doesn't really make sense because someone employed to answer calls can do that standing or sitting. An adjustment or accommodation could be to provide a stool, seating, or an adopted workspace, or using assistive technology for support

'MUST BE ABLE TO TYPE'

If your role requirements are stating a person must be able to type, you have automatically ruled out those who do not or cannot use a keyboard. This will inadvertently disqualify this individual. An adjustment or accommodation would instead be opting for text-to-speech software. Instead, you opt for something neutral, such as 'data entry' or 'data input required'. There is more than one way to interact with a computer, and assistive technology supports with that.

'MUST BE ABLE TO SEE, HEAR...'

Relying on words such as 'see' or 'hear' to define a task could also deter blind, d/Deaf, or hard of hearing individuals. When writing requirements, it is important to explain what the task is and make it clear to a candidate that alternatives are considered, otherwise telling someone they need to see to use a computer is ruling out that assistive technology we keep talking about. We always need to consider if an adjustment or accommodation can be made.

We've put together some of the most commonly used role requirements that are inherently excluding Disabled people.

Get rid of	Replace with
'Must be able to see attention to detail'	'Attention to detail is required'
'Must listen to instruction carefully'	'Must be able to communicate'
'Must be able to stand for long periods'	'Will require long periods of standing, with adjustments/accommodations provided'
'Must be energetic and active'	'The role will require some physical activity, with adjustments/accommodations available'
'Must be able to drive'	'This role will involve travel, with adjustments/accommodations available'
'Must be able to type'	'This role will require data entry, with adjustments/accommodations available'
'Must be able to work under pressure'	'The role will involve working in stressful environments. Support and adjustments/accommodations are available'

cont.

Get rid of	Replace with
'Must have a clear speaking voice'	'This role involves communicating verbally; however, alternative communication styles may be considered'
'Must be able to lift'	'This role involves physical tasks which will require lifting etc. Adjustments/accommodations may be considered'
'Must be able to work long hours'	'This role may require working overtime; flexible working hours or adjustments/accommodations are available'
'Must be able to multitask'	'This role involves managing multiple tasks at once. Adjustments/accommodations are available'
'Must be able to work in a fast-paced environment'	'This role involves working in a dynamic work environment, with adjustments/accommodations available'

IS A DEGREE ACTUALLY NEEDED?

For some Disabled people, obtaining a degree is unachievable due to lack of support, funding, accessibility, and so on. This may mean we do not have the qualifications organisations seem to want for every single role. Not only is this requirement inequitable for Disabled people who have not had the privilege of education, it has the potential to exclude people from underrepresented socio-economic backgrounds. We cannot assume every person has a degree.

The education system is not the most inclusive space. It supports the neuro-majority and the non-Disabled. It supports those who can navigate the world without access needs, adjustments, or accommodations. So please stop asking for a degree for every single role, especially for entry level roles, unless it is actually relevant, like a graduate role.

Role requirements wield a lot of influence on whether a Disabled candidate will proceed or not. Make it clear that adjustments and accommodations are considered, and that you are flexible. By making changes to your role requirements, removing the 'nice to haves' and actually focusing on the essentials needed, you can begin to create a more attractive and inviting role for a Disabled candidate. By promoting adjustments and accommodations you can help remove the stigma and fear a Disabled candidate might have. You reassure a candidate that you are open to treating them in an equitable manner and you demonstrate that you understand that not every person navigates the recruitment process in the same way.

Writing anti-ableist job descriptions

Your job descriptions have the potential to exclude Disabled people from the offset, so that's why when crafting them your hiring teams need to be adequately trained on how to communicate in an inclusive, anti-ableist way. Let's look at how we can make these more welcoming for Disabled candidates.

REMOVE THE ACRONYMS AND JARGON

Yes, it might take you less time to write a few letters as opposed to a whole group of words, or to use industry-specific jargon rather than dissect its meaning, but to anyone unaware or unfamiliar with that jargon or acronym, it's unclear. For example, DEI could translate as Diversity Ends Inclusion to someone unaware that it actually stands for, diversity, equity, and inclusion, and with this current climate, is that really a message you want to mis-communicate?

You can't assume that everyone is aware of the meaning of every acronym. You also need to consider that acronyms can mean different things across different industries. When a job description is filled with acronyms and jargon, it doesn't make for clear reading, and if someone is using a screen reader, it might mispronounce an acronym, making it difficult to understand. For example, 'NHS' might be read as 'nuhs' instead of 'N-H-S'. And honestly, it just sounds as if you're using fancy words to say something that could have been said in a much more effective way.

Here's an example of a jargon-ridden job description: 'Seeking a proactive SME to optimise KPIs working with SLAs to ensure alignment with OKRs, CFs, and PIs in a fast-paced B2B & B2C environment.' It looks as if someone pulled letters out of a scrabble game and flung them at a job description! Even writing it was confusing. Now imagine how this sounds to a person new to an industry, using a screen reader or who is dyslexic? You've created a scrabble of inaccessibility.

Instead try: 'We are looking for an experienced [insert subject] expert to improve performance metrics, support service agreements, and ensure our goals are met. You will be working with both business to business and consumer to consumer.' This is so much clearer, and it tells a candidate what they will actually be doing. It should not take a person asking their friends, mum, dad, granny's uncle to understand what you mean.

Promote flexibility

No, we don't mean do the splits; we mean understand that candidates might need:

- an alternative way to communicate
- the interview questions ahead of time
- extra time to complete a task

- time off for medical appointments
- remote working
- flexible working arrangements.

Not every Disabled person can work in an office. Some offices are not accessible, and some are just sensory overload waiting to happen. It's for that reason we need to push away from a return to the office. Covid-19 showed the world that we can work remotely; in fact, Disabled people were doing this long before the pandemic.

Being flexible means being accommodating to a colleague who has a flare up and can't work from the office one day. It might mean creating a quiet space within the office for neurodivergent colleagues to find some peace and balance. It could also mean understanding that what a Disabled person is able to do day to day, might not be the same every day.

Not everyone thrives in the hustle and bustle of a busy loud office. Some people find it much more productive to work from home, able to control the environments around them. Being flexible means being open to providing adjustments and accommodations that promote flexible working. Promoting flexible working in your job descriptions means you need to also follow this through. We are looking at you, those organisations who promise flexible working but don't allow it for the first year, the first three months – that is not flexible working; that is dangling a carrot.

Include a point of contact

Provide a point of contact to support a person with any questions or concerns or if they want to discuss the role requirements. And yes, your recruiter may find themselves at the receiving end of more questions, but isn't it a testament to a candidate who is asking the questions? This candidate who has envisioned themselves working for you and is going out of their way to learn more. While you might worry about extra messages coming through, this is where setting clear expectations for the point of contact is useful:

> If you require any adjustments/accommodations during the application process, please contact [email address]. This inbox is solely for discussing adjustments/accommodations; general recruitment queries should be directed to [another contact or careers page].

You can also consider an online submission form!

Add an inclusion statement, but actually be doing the work

An inclusive statement typically reads something along the lines of, 'We welcome applications from diverse backgrounds, communities' or, 'We particularly welcome applications from XYZ minority groups.' These statements are meant to reassure an individual that an organisation welcomes them, but the reality is they are empty promises of inclusion, unless you are doing the work both internally and externally. If and when you have begun to create an inclusive, anti-ableist culture, you should promote that.

Your inclusion statement needs to be evidenced in your recruitment process. By creating an inclusive job description, an equitable interviewing process, and an accessible onboarding process, you are living up to that inclusive statement. You are showing that you do welcome Disabled candidates. You are showing that you understand the inclusion you are preaching about. An inclusive statement can be reassuring when it is evidenced and felt across your recruitment process. When you are able to back up your inclusive statement with evidenced action, you no longer are talking the talk, but walking the walk.

Provide next steps

Providing information about the next steps provides clarity and reassurance for any candidate. For those of us who are neurodivergent, for example, not knowing what's next can leave us feeling anxious.

Providing these next steps and estimated timelines can do wonders for a person. Value your candidate's time and they will feel it; they will want to apply even more. Treat them as a number or as disposable and they will know it. They will feel it. No one likes waiting, so clarity on next steps and timescales is an inclusive step for everyone.

An inclusive, ableist free job description is not the whole answer; it is merely one spoke on the wheel. One piece of the puzzle. One step to creating a recruitment process that is anti-ableist.

Sourcing Disabled talent

Not every job board or platform is accessible or usable for Disabled people. When posting an opportunity/open role this should be done using multiple channels. Both the UK and US governments agree on the importance of using multiple channels to recruit Disabled individuals. The UK Government's guidance on inclusive communication highlights that utilising a variety of channels, such as mainstream media, Disability-specific publications, and organisational networks, is crucial for effectively reaching Disabled audiences (Disability Office, 2021). By broadening your recruitment channels and working with Disability organisations, you increase the chance of attracting the right talent and creating a truly inclusive workforce (UK Government, 2023).

Be sure to utilise Disability-specific job boards, job boards that support Disabled talent, such as Evenbreak, a global Disability job board which matches Disabled talent to inclusive employers. Other job boards include AbilityJOBS, Disability Solutions Career Centre, or Jobs4Disability. You could also partner with local Disability charities and NGOs to create new talent pools while making a difference by supporting local communities.

While there are also lots of Disabled groups, networks, and communities online out there that your teams could source Disabled talent from, we recommend that if you're using these, you do so respectfully, ask permission to post open roles, and don't spam groups.

Applications

Let's be honest, recruitment hasn't really changed that much over the last few decades. Yes, we have moved away from relying on paper applications, but we are still relying on an application of some sort to be completed. We still rely on a CV or a person submitting a completed form. If you rely on a webpage application, you need to be sure that the page is accessible. This means ensuring it is usable and has points of contact to request support if needed. The page must be accessible for people using assistive technology. But what if we were to suggest that you could look at alternatives to just a form or CV submission?

We encourage organisations to be creative, to be flexible with their applications. Don't just ask a person to complete a form; offer alternative formats to apply. Consider video CVs or video applications, email applications, and even over-the-phone applications.

It is likely that your current application process was designed without consideration or understanding of accessibility. Recognise the various needs of individuals.

Candidate self-identifies or asks for an adjustment/accommodation

Disability is not something to fear. In fact, you don't even need to know if someone is Disabled. But if you do have the privilege of having someone share their Disability with you, or they do ask for adjustments and accommodations, your response could either make or break their willingness to continue an application. It could affect their internalised ableism. A response such as, 'You don't look Disabled' or, 'I would never have known' will only make visible your own ableism. It demonstrates your lack of awareness and training. It's a big red flag that tells a person that your organisation is not the one for them. Don't assume our needs, but create an environment that is welcoming and open. Don't fear us; we're already potentially fearing the what ifs of our application, so help us remove that fear. Understand that every person, Disabled or not, has individual access needs.

We need you to be open and empathetic and to understand that us sharing our lived experience or requesting adjustments and accommodations takes a lot at times. If and when a person does share with you, thank them, acknowledge it, and ask, 'Is there anything I can do to make the process more accessible', or ask if they require an adjustment or accommodation to support them through this process.

Do not be the reason we withdraw. Do not be the reason we leave this recruitment process feeling defeated, yet again.

Candidate screening and selection

Your hiring teams need to understand the importance of reviewing CVs without bias. They need to be able to assess a candidate's suitability for a role without making an ableist assumption simply because the candidate self-identified or asked for the questions ahead of time.

When hiring teams make assumptions, they are allowing their bias to interject. One of the biggest assumptions made by hiring teams is that a candidate with gaps on their CV or with short employment periods is not loyal and cannot hold down a job. This assumption, of course, completely neglects the difficulties Disabled people face when struggling to gain and retain employment.

Being hired is only one piece of a bigger picture. And of course, Disabled people have gaps in their CVs. As you are learning, we don't even get a chance to apply before we are faced with one ableist barrier after another. So please stop judging us for our employment history. Be open to the fact that not everyone has had the privilege of working five or more years for the same company. For some of us, having a job for longer than a few months has been a win.

Within employment, many Disabled people will face challenges when receiving adjustments and accommodations, with some being dismissed for attendance due to sick days while waiting for adjustments and accommodations to arrive. Trust us, we have been there. So yes, we might not always have the longest employment stints or we might have gaps on our CV, but we are so much more than our past experiences and trauma.

Candidate selection should not take into consideration us self-identifying or us asking for an adjustment or accommodation. That is illegal. That is discrimination. But that unfortunately is the reason some of us have never heard back from your hiring teams, only we don't get told it's because we are Disabled; it's that there was a better fit for the role. Or it's just radio silence as a recruiter suddenly goes cold and ghosts us.

It is so important that hiring teams making the decisions should be receiving bias intervention training, helping them to understand the bias that is ingrained in us all. This training should also focus on ableism and support hiring teams to unlearn the ableism in their actions. This training should not be a one-off either. It should be updated and revised annually.

Interviewing

Much like candidate selection, interviewing has the potential to allow a recruiter to inadvertently perpetuate ableism. We recommend that organisations have their hiring teams read our language chapter, which explores language and the ableism ingrained in people's responses when presented with or discussing Disability.

When offering interviews, it is important to be as flexible as possible. Not every candidate will succeed during an in-person meeting; for example, there might be bright lights causing issues for their focus, or the office the interview is being held in may be loud, or the building is not accessible, so the candidate had no choice but to request a virtual interview. Remember, the world is not designed for us.

Barriers to in-person interviews

Organisations fail to audit and measure how accessible their offices are, and when a Disabled candidate with mobility access needs arrives for an interview, they can find themselves unable to attend because the lift is out of service or because the floor did not have enough space to move freely. Now imagine a role requirement was to be in office and this Disabled person showed up each day after being employed only to face the same broken lift? Does that seem fair or equitable to you?

Here are some other barriers they might face:

- **Physical barriers:** Such as not being able to get to the location, the office not being accessible, or there is no accessible parking.

- **Sensory barriers:** Such as harsh or flickering lighting in interview space or background noise which is overwhelming and makes it hard to hear.

- **Communication barriers:** Such as interviewer using unclear language, not being offered a sign language interpreter, or lack of clarity by interviewer when asking questions.

- **Bias:** Such as an interviewer making assumptions about a candidate's Disability or making judgements about their capability based on their Disability alone.

Prior to conducting interviews, offer a choice of in-person or virtual meeting. Know the accessibility of the interview location and what is and is not possible. Always – and we mean always – ask a candidate if they require any adjustments or accommodations prior to any interview and be sure to follow through with implementing them.

Ableist bias during interviews

When conducting an interview, hiring teams need to stop passing judgement on a person's body language. Let's explore this in more detail.

Bias	Bias unpacked
Not maintaining eye contact	Maintaining eye contact can be uncomfortable or even painful for visually impaired, blind, or neurodivergent candidates.
Slow or delayed response	A slower response time could be due to cognitive differences, neurodivergence, or brain injury. It does not mean the candidate is incapable but rather needs the time to process.

Unusual body language	People with sensory processing issues or anxiety might move their bodies to help self-regulate (stim).
Asking for clarity	Asking repeated questions for clarity may help someone with a learning Disability or neurodivergence to process information in a more digestible way.
Unusual speaking style	Some candidates who stutter, speak with an accent, or use a speech device may be perceived as less articulate or capable. However, this does not make them less articulate or capable.

When interviewing you should be interviewing for the skills and experiences required for the role. Adding additional ableist requirements about a person's body language just sets Disabled people up to fail. Be flexible during the interview, encourage the candidate to take some time before answering a question, and maybe even go a step further and provide the interview questions ahead of time.

Creating equitable interviews

You can offer all candidates the opportunity to receive interview questions ahead of time. The purpose of an interview is to get the best out of a person. By creating an equitable experience your hiring teams can help support someone to bring their best, and we also have to remember that it is not just the candidate being interviewed; the organisation is being interviewed by the candidate. This means your hiring teams need to be able to provide a welcoming space, which is supportive, responsive, and provides equitable opportunities.

When we say responsive, we mean that hiring teams need to follow up where they have said they would. They need to implement any accessibility requests and use a candidate's preferred communication style. Be sure your hiring teams are telling candidates about any employee networks/groups and diversity, equity, and inclusion initiatives within your organisation.

We all want to know who it is we are going to be working for. Providing information on these groups shows your commitment to creating an inclusive and representative culture. It can help make a candidate feel represented and it can reassure them that other Disabled people work here too.

So, tell candidates about these groups. Add information to your website. Add it to marketing content, include it in the job spec. Shout or sign it from the rooftop. Make sure your recruiters can answer questions about the culture, accessibility, and the adjustments and accommodations process. Remember that your organisation is being interviewed by us as much as you are interviewing us.

> 66 It's very natural, and perfectly understandable, for recruiters and hiring managers to feel a bit nervous around hiring Disabled people. What if you say the 'wrong' thing, or unintentionally offend someone? How do you offer the right support, when you know very little about Disability? What happens if you've never heard of the condition a candidate has?
>
> Thankfully, there is no need to worry. Recruiters and hiring managers aren't expected to be experts on every medical condition or diagnosis. In fact, the name of the condition is irrelevant. What is relevant are the barriers the Disabled candidate might face in the recruitment process, or the role itself, and what you can do to remove them. Say, for example, a candidate tells you they have a condition called spondylolisthesis.

That information is of little value to you. However, if they tell you that they are unable to stand for long, and will need to mostly sit, you can discuss if or how the job may be adapted to a seating position. If a candidate tells you they have dyslexia, again, that's not really helpful. Every person with dyslexia will face different barriers and need different adjustments. If they tell you they would prefer information in short paragraphs or bullet points, rather than large blocks of text, that is information you can use.

The main requirement for a hiring manager or recruiter isn't an encyclopaedic knowledge of medical conditions. It's the ability to ask the question, 'What barriers might you face, and what can I do to ensure this process works for you?' Then it's simply a case of listening to the answer, and having a conversation about what is possible. The Disabled person will be the expert in what they require, so you don't need to be. 99

– Jane Hatton, CEO and Founder of Evenbreak

Building anti-ableist workplaces

Workplaces are built on the inaccessible blocks of exclusion. Disability is not represented within leadership or management and outdated policies and processes create one inaccessible barrier after another.

We often find that organisations start with recruitment, believing that simply hiring Disabled people is the answer, when the fact is, hiring Disabled people is not enough. Organisations need to be able to develop us, promote us, and retain us. Failing to create a welcoming, accessible workplace is not going to make a new joiner or an existing colleague feel any sense of belonging. If we are having to experience challenges daily or facing barriers and red tape when trying to acquire adjustments and accommodations and some form of equitable support, we are going to mask. We are going to withdraw, and we are not going to feel valued.

Organisations fear Disability and they fear the consequence of getting it wrong, of breaking the law. But Disabled people do not want to be having to threaten organisations with legal action and we do not want to be discriminated against, we do not want to be excluded. We understand that there are going to be mistakes and a lack of understanding along the way. What we need most from you is to be open to learning. Be open to making change once you learn.

So, let's look at how you can unlearn the ableism ingrained in an organisation's workplace culture.

66 Unlearning ableism in the workplace means unlearning the beliefs that Disabled needs are special needs, that accommodations or adjustments are special treatment, and that a Disability indicates a lack of competence or capability.

Disabled employees have the same needs as all employees. They need an effective way to apply, to showcase their skills and abilities in interviews, and the technology, training, and leadership to do their job once hired. The tech team needs different training and technology than the marketing team, who needs different supports than the finance team, and so on. Basic human needs are the same; it is how those needs must be met that differs.

Accommodations and accommodating aren't specific to the Disability community, but basic tenets of being human. When we ask for someone to give us directions or to withhold a certain ingredient, or we tell them that we will be late, we are asking for an accommodation. Every product, service, or feature ever created is an accommodation – a solution designed to meet a specific need.

Disabled people aren't being hired or promoted less because they are less capable, but because they are judged as less capable. If somebody is seen as competent and capable until they disclose their Disability, it's not the Disability that is the problem; it's the judgement of it.

In summary, Disabilities are a natural variation of being human. Disability needs are human needs. Accommodations are basic tenets of being human. And if someone has to hide their Disability to be respected, accepted, or hired, the problem isn't the Disability, but the judgement of it. 99

– **Julie Harris, Disability inclusion activist, speaker, and author** of *Boldly Belong: The Power of Being You in a Disabling Society*

Training

Disability training in the workplace often focuses on the 'risks' of hiring Disabled people or not providing support. 'If we don't provide adjustments, they will sue us.' 'If we say the wrong thing, they will sue us.' 'Disabled people are so expensive.' These are real thoughts people have when they do not receive adequate Disability training in the workplace.

Trainers educating about Disability but not having the lived experience or acquired knowledge of the subject is not adequate. Nor is training that fails to centre the human behind the lived experience, the people behind the Disability, which, as we are learning in this book, is essential if we are ever to unlearn ableism.

Yes, the vast majority of workplace Disability training fails to address ableism, accessibility, intersectionality, or internalised ableism. In fact, 94.3% of Disabled people feel there is not enough being done to address ableism in the workplace (Disabled by Society, 2024). So how do we make training anti-ableist?

Organisations should be working with Disabled-led organisations, charities, and Disabled consultants to create bespoke human-centric training that goes beyond legal compliance and obligations, training that does not shy away from teaching people about ableism, accountability, accessibility, and allyship. We need training that is being delivered by the people who get it, because they have been through it – people who understand Disability.

This training should not be a one-off thing either. All employees within an organisation should have ableism and accessibility training as part of their onboard training, as well as the organisation's workplace adjustment and accommodation process.

Specific training should also be delivered for different departments and roles; for example, people managers should have training on supporting colleagues during the workplace adjustment and accommodation process, recruitment teams on how to make the recruitment process accessible, marketing teams on how to create accessible content, and so on. But before creating any training you need to make it accessible.

Prior to training

- Create the training in various formats. For example, if you have training which is live on teams, make sure you can record this, caption it, create a transcript, and share it on your internal learning platform.

- Consider the accessibility of the platforms you use when delivering virtual training. Can the platform provide captions? Is there a chat functionality? Is the platform usable if a person has their screen zoomed in?

- Follow universal design principles by adding alt text, checking colour contrast, inserting captions for videos, and so on. Following these principles can help open up the training to a wider audience.

- Represent Disability in any imagery or video – and by represent we do not mean a white wheelchair user.

- Be sure trainers have their own training on supporting diverse learning needs and communicating accessibly.

Delivering training

- Before any training, send an agenda along with your accessibly designed slide deck. This creates equity by allowing everyone to follow along at their own pace and reduces the burden someone may have felt if they had to ask for the deck by means of an adjustment or accommodation.

- When delivering the training, it is important not to miss information from the slides you are using. Be sure to talk through any imagery and graphics. Don't assume everyone can see your slides and don't assume everyone learns in the same way.

- Schedule breaks regularly to accommodate various learning paces.

- If delivering training virtually, be sure to allow people the option to leave their camera on or off. Not everyone benefits from being on camera, as some people find it an overwhelming distraction or can't see what's on the screen.

- Engage with your audience, ask questions, and always ask if they need adjustments or accommodations or if there is a more accessible way for them to participate.

- Gather feedback from those in attendance to improve on their experiences.

Ableism needs to be part of your training right from day one; colleagues need to be aware of your company stance on ableist behaviours, and they need to feel safe in your workplace.

Training needs to stop reducing Disability to a risk, and instead create a person-centred, diverse syllabus which covers ableism, accessibility, adjustments and accommodations, allyship, intersectionality, and the diversity of Disability. The training needs to be mandatory for every colleague. In fact, your hiring teams and people managers should have additional training which focuses more on facilitating conversations, addressing bias, and understanding specific adjustment and accommodation processes. Training needs to be fit for purpose, accessible, and reviewed and updated regularly. And if you need help with this, reach out to Disabled by Society, which supports organisations globally to transform Disability exclusion to inclusion, and helps change the way people think, learn about, and view Disability.

People managers

When starting any new role, it can feel overwhelming for a Disabled person. We are about to navigate an unknown environment, and many of us will be met with an all too familiar sense of fear. We fear self-identifying or asking for support, because for many of us the workplace has been a source of rejection and discrimination. According to Evenbreak (Hatton, 2020), 71% of Disabled people rate employers poorly for their understanding of Disability, highlighting the need for organisations to do better, and this is where we feel people managers can play a fundamental role.

People managers can create an environment where we want to show up, where we feel safe to self-identify, and where we can ask for support, get it and not be ignored. But many of us fear the response from our manager:

- Will they know the adjustment and accommodation process?

- Will they treat me differently?

- Will they begin to speak to me in a different tone of voice, act strangely, or tiptoe around me?

- Will there be radio silence? Will they ignore me?

Self-identifying or asking for support in the workplace and opening up to a manager takes strength and courage. It's not easy to ask when in the past that request has been ignored. Many of us have found that when we share information, our managers haven't exactly been supportive and they haven't exactly been open to learning. The Great Big Workplace Adjustments Survey (Business Development Forum, 2023) revealed that 56% of Disabled employees continued to face Disability-related barriers in the workplace even after adjustments were made. Additionally, only 18% felt that the adjustments they received had removed all barriers, and just 10% found it easy to obtain the adjustments they needed.

Further research by Deloitte (2024) highlighted that over 40% of Disabled employees reported experiencing discrimination from their managers or co-workers, with many citing a lack of understanding and support when discussing their needs. People managers, it's time to stop fearing Disability, it's time to stop burying your heads in the sand. Below are some suggestions for what you should do.

Educate yourself

Make a conscious effort to learn about Disability, both visible and non-visible. Attend trainings, do some of your own research. Read, listen to audio books, or if a colleague in your team shares what their Disability is, do some homework so that you can have conversations which can help you provide better support. Always take a lead from the individual.

See the individual

Treat your team members as individuals. Not every flower thrives with the same amount of water or sunlight. Some need shade, some need darkness. Your team have different needs, some of us have access needs, some of us need you to communicate more clearly, or provide questions and agendas ahead of time. But most of all, what we need is a manager who listens, who lets us lead the conversation, but then leads us to the resources and helps us through the process; a manager who we can be open with, can share, can offload to; a manager who goes beyond managing, and leads.

Don't label

Labelling a person as 'difficult' because they have had to ask for support, or in most cases, have had to chase their manager multiple times in order to receive support, is a slap in the face. But it is the harsh reality for many Disabled people. Colleagues who need clarity, colleagues who need to ask questions, colleagues who are not able to read between the lines are all too easily labelled as difficult, when underneath these dismissive attitudes of managers is laziness. They are often too lazy to take the time to support, too lazy to care, too lazy to take accountability, and too lazy to lead.

Know the adjustment and accommodation process

People managers should be setting the bar for others, showing them by example how to support Disabled workers. When people managers are not familiar with the adjustment and accommodation process they are unable to provide any kind of reassurance to a Disabled employee, which in turn causes instability for that employee. Not knowing this process can create unnecessary delays, causing the employee to potentially take additional time off. Better to be in employment struggling, than searching for employment as a Disabled person. That's the thinking many of us have when we are in roles with unsupportive managers, who have not been adequately trained and who, when we do push back and ask why there are delays, label us as 'difficult'.

Create an open space

Create a space where team members can approach you to ask for support or workplace adjustments and accommodations. When a Disabled team member shares with you, don't make assumptions, listen to what they have to say; don't make empty promises, or become defensive. Really listen so that you can understand.

Be flexible

Offer employees flexibility, whether it is working hours, working remotely, taking time off for medical appointments, or even if it is extra time for a task. Understand and recognise the individual's needs.

Be reactive, not responsive

Anyone can manage, but it takes a different kind of person to lead, and it takes a leader to be able to say, 'I don't know the answer right now, but let me get it and get back to you within a day.' This is a manager who is reactive not responsive, who understands that to get the best out of people you have to treat people as people. This is a manager who doesn't start to treat you differently when they find out you're Disabled.

Provide equitable career opportunities

Don't overlook Disabled people for promotions or career development. We want to succeed, we want to develop, we want to have an equitable opportunity to do so. This also includes performance reviews. Be sure when completing performance reviews that you are taking account of a person's Disability. For example, if someone is being scored on verbal communication but they are non-verbal, take into account their communication style, which might be written. Measuring Disabled people against non-Disabled people without taking into account adjustments and accommodations and the barriers Disabled employees have to experience will exclude us.

Lead by example

If you use ableist humour or make derogatory comments about a person's Disability, you are creating an unsafe environment and setting an example of ableism for your team. Challenge ableism in the moment; don't say anything or laugh along. You need to lead by example and show your team that you don't tolerate ableism and that your work environment is a safe, welcoming space for everyone.

Create an anti-ableist policy

Anti-ableist policies create an environment in which Disabled colleagues can feel psychologically safe, where we can self-identify without fear of consequence or discrimination, and where equity and inclusion are more than mere words but cemented in your foundations. Establish a zero-tolerance policy on ableism. This means defining what ableism is, providing examples of ableist behaviours and language. Be sure to add a process for reporting ableist experiences confidentially.

This anti-ableist policy should be clear and accessible for everyone, as should all your policies. That includes adjustments and accommodations policies which provide timeframes, points of contact, and alternative ways to escalate if needed. Policies need to go beyond what the law says. They need to go beyond the 'legal language' of Disability.

We cannot expect to create inclusive workplaces if our policies were written during the dawn of floppy disks. (A floppy disk was a little disk used to save and transport data from one computer to another.)

Policies need to be updated and reviewed regularly. They should take into account feedback from Disabled colleagues or/and external Disability consultants. The language used should reflect your organisation's commitment to inclusion, accessibility, and equity. Learn more about policy and ableism in Chapter 8.

> 66 Disability groups are often referred to as a Disability and neurodiversity network, employee resource group (ERG), or community. These groups help to create a sense of community for Disabled and neurodivergent people in the workplace. They should be Disabled-led, ensuring it is Disabled people's voices being heard and represented, but open to everyone to join and learn how to better support and act as an ally. An organisation should be ensuring leadership buy-in and support for such a group. Who better to know how inclusive an organisation is than those who know the good, the bad, and the inaccessible? Those who have experienced it. These communities can become a

critical friend to an organisation, helping to elevate and amplify Disabled voices.

ERGs are a valuable resource for organisations to create communities and help employees feel a sense of belonging in the workplace. But their impact goes far beyond the communities they're built for.

It's that thing of, 'you don't know what you don't know'. Typically, unless you identify with specific communities, you aren't exposed to conversations around such topics. ERGs can create safe spaces to share, discuss, and learn about topics which might otherwise feel uncomfortable, and this enables everyone to be part of the conversation.

I have learned a lot about myself through joining an ERG, initially as an ally. I was exposed to conversations that I had never heard before; I was able to listen to people with direct lived experience, and I was able to understand beyond what I unconsciously grew up believing, or what society had me believe.

I learned I was AuDHD (autistic and ADHD) at the age of 28. Although an ERG isn't a diagnostic tool, if it wasn't for an ERG, and never being exposed to these types of conversations, I would never have known.

So, as much as they create communities and foster belonging in the workplace, they go far beyond the communities they are built for.

If you're an organisation and you haven't got an ERG – why not? 99

**– David Shiels, AuDHD, global Disability
and neurodiversity lead**

Leadership buy-in

Encourage leadership teams to work collaboratively with Disability groups and networks that you have established. It is all well and good to say you're an inclusive organisation but if your leaders haven't got the foggiest idea of allyship or aren't able to talk about Disability without doing so in a condescending, ableist way, then they need to do better. Your leadership teams should be buying into your Disability inclusion.

Embed accessibility across your organisation

Your company branding, your brand colours, your training, your onboarding, your anything and everything designed have the potential to create disabling inaccessible barriers. Most organisations have never considered accessibility as part of the initial design process. It was and is still very much seen as an added extra, an additional step, a forced step because organisations don't want to break the law. Because accessibility has not been at the forefront of designing workplaces, inaccessible ablist barriers have been erected across every area of your business. Accessibility is not just the responsibility of one team or one person, but rather the responsibility of your entire organisation. Accessible design should be part of your processes for everything, from marketing, recruitment, human resources, branding, communication team, and so on. Read more about accessibility in Chapter 9.

Representing Disability

In marketing, content, and media: Spoiler, you won't ever represent every Disabled person. There's no way to do that unless you somehow magically managed to cram every single Disabled person on the planet into one image. That's never going to happen, and you would also need a really wide lens. When choosing imagery to represent Disability, use authentic images. Stop using the same stock imagery that everyone else is using. Take your own pictures. It tells a truthful story, that actual people who are Disabled work here. Ask your colleagues to get involved, ask your Disability employee resource groups and networks to get involved. But always get consent and do not pressure anyone into saying yes. Show people using adjustments and accommodations. Include images of people with stimming aids. Equally, include images of any sensory rooms or quiet spaces you've designed in the office. Show the accessible environments you are creating. Demonstrate to candidates that you are an organisation that considers Disability, that represents Disability.

In leadership: Of course, your marketing is only one area of representation. Your organisation needs to represent Disability across your executive and leadership teams. Again, we know Disability is not always visible and we cannot force a person to self-identify at work, but by creating spaces that are inclusive and accessible we encourage colleagues to put themselves out there, to succeed, to feel a sense of belonging. The US Bureau of Labor Statistics (2024) reports that Disabled individuals are underrepresented in management, professional, and related occupations. In 2023, only 37.4% of Disabled workers held jobs in these fields, compared to 43.9% of non-Disabled workers, highlighting that Disabled people are not being represented in leadership positions, which often can leave them unheard and unseen. By removing the ableist barriers we provide the opportunity for Disabled people to succeed.

Read more about representation in Chapter 10.

Making adjustment processes accessible!

Your adjustment and accommodation process needs to be fit for purpose. A person waiting three months for a screen reader is not fit for purpose. The process should not solely rely on us speaking to a manager and telling them we are struggling; there should be alternative options for colleagues to request adjustments and accommodations. There should be:

- a policy to support and provide reassurance, timelines, and guidance

- a point of contact for further questions or escalations if required

- accountability from your leadership and people managers to know and understand any adjustments and accommodations policies and process.

Adjustments and accommodations can empower and give support, and they make a difference to our confidence and our ability to succeed. Provide examples of what can be offered. Provide a list of commonly requested adjustments and accommodations and be sure that if a person is requesting them, they are given timescales and follow-up responses, and are not being asked to prove they are Disabled. Yes, you heard that right, some organisations ask for proof of Disability before providing adjustments and accommodations. Unless your team are medical professionals then checking for proof of someone's Disability will always be beyond their professional skills. Adjustments and accommodations are about providing equitable support. Equity should not come with the requirement of proof.

Remember, it is a legal requirement in many countries to provide workplace adjustments and accommodations.

Develop us

A study by Deloitte (2024) found that 28% of Disabled people reported being passed over for promotion. But it shouldn't surprise you to learn that Disabled people have aspirations just like everyone else. Don't just hire us under some intern programme that only lasts two weeks; offer us real roles, with growth and development. We want meaningful employment; we told you already you need to be doing more than hiring Disabled people! You need to be developing us, promoting us, and creating equitable opportunities for us to get there.

When it comes to performance reviews and performance plans, organisations need to rethink the way they review and measure colleagues against each other.

- Using verbal communication as a performance metric unfairly disadvantages a person who is unable or struggles to verbally communicate.

- Using speed of task completion as a performance metric can unfairly disadvantage someone who is methodical and detail oriented.

- Expecting constant participation in meetings can overlook those who contribute meaningfully to written formats instead.

- Measuring success by visibility in the workplace can under-value remote workers or those who work best independently.

- Judging leadership potential based on extroversion can exclude highly effective but introverted leaders.

Using a rigid one-size-fits-all approach to productivity can fail to account for different working styles of Disabled and neurodivergent individuals. Focus on the individual and identify any possible ableism or inaccessible barriers that could restrict the opportunity.

- **Understand individual needs:** Ask how we work best rather than assuming a standard approach, ask about adjustments and accommodations, review current adjustments and accommodations and their suitability for the role.

- **Provide flexibility:** We have said it once and we will say it again.

- **Eliminate barriers:** Identify and remove inaccessible tools, spaces, or expectations.

- **Listen and collaborate:** Involve Disabled and neurodivergent individuals in decision-making; don't make decisions for us, without us.

- **Respect different workflows:** Allow for varied pacing, breaks, or assistive technologies.

- **Challenge ableism:** Question productivity norms that prioritise speed over sustainability.

Even having a role or working in an organisation doesn't mean a Disabled person is safe. During times of lay-offs and redundancies, Disabled people are often some of the first to go. Disabled people deserve the same respect as our non-Disabled peers in the workplace; we deserve to be valued just as much, and we should have the same opportunities as everybody else.

Organisations have a long way to go to in unlearning ableism. It is not something that is going to change overnight; it will take months and years. Some organisations will be much further ahead than others, and some will just be starting. Unlearning the ableism in your recruitment and cultures is not the answer – it is only the start. It is the start of taking accountability. It is establishing an accessibility roadmap, helping you to plan ahead, encouraging you to ask the questions, 'Where are we now?', 'Where do we need to be?' and 'How do we get there?'

No matter your starting point, a starting point is needed. Put your money where your mouth is. No more talking the talk of inclusion. It is time to actually unlearn the ableism in our recruitment and workplace cultures.

CHAPTER 13
Unlearning Ableism:
Health and Social Care

> **Doctor, I feel as if you're not listening to me. Nurse, I know my body. Care worker, I can hear what you are saying; I'm sitting right here. Just because I'm Disabled doesn't mean you know me better than I know myself. For the love of health and social care, show me you actually care!**

Health and social care systems are injected with a medical model view of Disability (medical pun!).

For Disabled people, this means we are often left experiencing the ableism of those who are meant to be supporting or taking care of us: doctors, nurses, care assistants, therapists, dentists, and so on. Although they can have the best intentions, these healthcare professions often just aren't aware of the ableism they are contributing to.

That's if a Disabled person can even make it through the front doors to meet them, because heaven forbid if a Disabled person visits a doctor or therapist's office and it be accessible (a rarity for many).

That's if they're even made aware they had an appointment, because, surprise, a lot of communication with Disabled patients or service users is inaccessible and completely neglects their access needs.

If a Disabled person does somehow overcome the inaccessible barriers prior to appointments, they then have ableist bias, stereotypes, and a medical model view of what it means to be Disabled to deal with.

Oh, what joy it is to be a Disabled person navigating the health and social care systems across society. But have no fear, we are going to turn the temperature down on ableism in health and social care!

Health and social care and the medical model of Disability

Whether you are born Disabled or acquired a Disability, you will inevitably spend some time getting tested and diagnosed, attending check-ups, seeing specialists, attending therapy and rehabilitation, requesting medical evidence, going to repeat visits, follow-up appointments, and so on. You are going to have spent, or will spend, some time getting up close and personal with health and social care. Unfortunately for us, health and social care systems are typically rooted in a medical model view of Disability.

Surprise, a medical model view of Disability in a medical setting – ironic, right?

This medical model view of Disability dominates across health and social care, shaping attitudes, behaviours, practices, treatment plans, and policies. Let's take a closer dive into what this undiagnosed ableism in health and social care settings has led to.

A focus on fixing or curing the Disabled person

The medical model of Disability prioritises treatment and 'fixing' a Disability, rather than considering accessibility, ableism, and the broader support needs of the individual. This can lead to healthcare professionals believing that a Disabled person's quality of life is inherently less, simply because they are Disabled, and thus they need to be 'fixed'. For example, imagine a person visiting the doctor with a chronic illness. They are seeking long-term support and a treatment plan, but instead, the doctor focuses only on fixing the pain in the short-term, offering only temporary pain relief and no consideration for sustainable, long-term support. This narrow approach can reinforce negative assumptions and ignore the social and environmental factors that affect Disabled people's well-being (European Parliament, 2020).

A view that Disabled lives are less valuable

The medical model view devalues Disabled people's lives as not being as valuable as non-Disabled people's. This can result in healthcare rationing, in which Disabled people are refused treatment. We only have to look at the Covid-19 pandemic for evidence of this, where Disabled people and elderly people were placed on Do Not Resuscitate (DNRs) orders without consent.

In the UK, the Care Quality Commission (2020) reported that over 500 care home residents were subjected to DNR orders without their consent during the pandemic. Disability rights organisations raised significant concerns about medical rationing protocols that could disproportionately impact Disabled individuals, potentially leading to the inappropriate application of DNR orders (Disability Rights Education and Defense Fund, 2020).

One-size-fits-all approaches, ignoring individual needs

The medical model of Disability reinforces a rigid one-size-fits-all approach to care, which overlooks accessibility. This means barriers for Disabled patients and service users. Think of a patient who is d/Deaf waiting to be called into an appointment. They are sat in the waiting area, but there lies a barrier. Each appointment is being called verbally, which means this d/Deaf person might struggle. Or consider a blind or visually impaired patient waiting to be called for an appointment. Rather than verbally calling the patient or service user when it is their turn, they use an automated signage, which flags up the patient's name – not very accessible for the blind or visually impaired person. Now imagine if this service provider used both a verbal cue and signage to make patients aware, offering alternatives for patients. Much better!

The King's Fund (Fenney, 2023) found that more than a third of healthcare professionals had never received any training on the Accessible Information Standard, a legal requirement for all NHS organisations in the UK since 2016. We have already mentioned accessibility loads, but it's important to reinforce. Accessibility is not just about patients entering the building; it's about how you communicate with us, how you support us, and how information is presented. We shouldn't have to fight for accessibility in healthcare settings, places you would expect to have a better understanding of the diverse needs of Disabled people.

Not listening to Disabled people

The medical model of Disability isn't known for taking its lead from Disabled people, you know, those people, the experts, with the actual lived experience. Instead, healthcare professionals often consider themselves the experts because they have medical training.

Think of a woman visiting a doctor who thinks she might be autistic. The doctor, on seeing she is verbal and articulates herself to a level they deem acceptable, disregards this patient's concerns because they don't fit the stereotype of what they believe autism to be, despite the doctor not being qualified in making an assessment. In fact, women often face delays in receiving autism diagnosis due to the historical view that autism is primarily a male condition, with diagnostic criteria and assessments being based on male presentations.

A 2025 study published in *The Journal of Child Psychology and Psychiatry* found that 54.2% of autistic females and 40.9% of autistic males received at least one psychiatric diagnosis before their autism diagnosis (Martini *et al.*, 2025). Not listening to Disabled patients and service users impacts care and will cause harm.

Quality of care

The medical model of Disability also impacts the care a patient or service user receives. It frames natural variations in human ability as medical problems, rather than as part of human diversity. In the past, this meant that many Disabled people were subjected to torture, pain, or humiliation as part of their treatment to 'fix' their Disability. Aversion therapy was used on Disabled children in the 1960s and 1970s, where they were subjected to painful stimuli such as electric shocks, used to 'correct' behaviour. Electroconvulsive therapy was used, particularly in the mid-20th century, on individuals labelled with 'mental Disabilities', often without consent, to 'treat' or 'control' behaviours (Wright, 2015).

Today, behaviour correction treatments are still prescribed. An example of this is Applied Behaviour Analysis (ABA) therapy. ABA therapy seeks to improve or modify specific behaviours through positive reinforcement. In literal terms, it means seeking to 'correct' or 'fix' an autistic person. Julia Bascom, Executive Director of Autistic Self Advocacy, says, 'The stated end goal of ABA is an autistic child who is "indistinguishable from their peers," an autistic child who can pass as neurotypical. We don't think that's an acceptable goal' (Bascom, 2019). The National Autistic Society (n.d.) also states that 'Autism is not something to be cured or fixed; it's a different way of being that brings both strengths and challenges.'

But yet these outdated practices of 'fixing' or making Disabled people comply to neurotypical or non-Disabled standards is evident within healthcare, with barbaric so-called treatments. An example of this is the Judge Rotenberg Center in the US, a residential facility known for its controversial use of aversive treatments, particularly electric skin shocks, as part of its behavior modification programme. These practices are used on people with intellectual and developmental Disabilities residing there. As of the time of this book being written, this is still happening, despite it being condemned by the United Nations as torture practices.

A social model informed treatment plan would include encouraging caregivers to create sensory friendly spaces, flexible routines, personalised support plans, speech and language therapy, augmentative communication devices, and so on. For caregivers, respite could also be a positive option. This social model informed approach is seeking to correct the environment, to enhance lives, rather than trying to fix or correct them, because, surprise, you can't cure autism.

The ableism in the waiting room

A study by the Urban Institute (Gonzalez et al., 2023) found that 32% of Disabled adults reported experiencing unfair treatment in a healthcare setting. That's nearly one in three Disabled people experiencing ableism, every time they visit a doctor, dentist, therapist, and so on. Let that sink in.

For many Disabled people, health and social care has left them feeling frustrated, anxious, and in a lot of ways let down by professionals:

- mistaking symptoms and blaming them on existing Disability

- falsely assuming that because a patient is fine one day, that they are getting better or are cured of their Disability

- having bias which delays diagnosis, because they believe that the patient does not fit their textbook example

- misdiagnosing conditions due to limited exposure to Disability

- not providing accessible ways for patients to communicate

- unaware of the bias they hold about Disability.

> 66 I approached my doctor to say that I felt I may have autism and/or ADHD, and I was prepared for a negative response. I wasn't prepared for the shady eye roll, the snigger, and the, 'I doubt that very much' response. Normally, this response could trigger me to explode into a sharp-tongued, verbal tirade of insults – my survival mode, for most of my teenage and adult life.
>
> I remained calm, gave them a well-documented list of reasons for thinking this, and asked for a referral for an assessment. 'Well, you've managed this far in life, so I don't see why you would need this diagnosis' was the response. This is where the shady, sarcastic David got to work. 'Oh, so finding myself in wild and dangerous situations as a teenager, just to try and fit in is managing life, is it?' 'Or do you think partying for days on end

just to try and escape the reality of my thoughts or feelings was managing?' 'What about being prescribed every antidepressant on the market because you fobbed it off as depression is managing?' I knew at this point I was on my own. I impulsively booked a private assessment, without a thought to the cost, as per usual. The outcome, as I expected, was that I have autism and ADHD.

So back to the eye rolling GP I went. This time, I had a bigger fight on my hands. Even though my diagnostic assessment was Gold Standard and met all the National Institute for Health and Care guidelines, I was told that it wouldn't be accepted by my local health trust and I would have to go on the waiting list to be assessed.

After four years of battling with various professionals, I finally got recognition of my diagnosis, but there currently was no support available in my area.

My story, unfortunately, is like thousands of others across the UK, who are being failed by a broken NHS system, battling with health professionals who have limited knowledge of autism or ADHD, and who are forced to pay for expensive diagnostic assessments, in the hope of professional support, with nothing at the other end. 〝

– David Johnston, 45-year-old AuDHD male

The inequity of global health and social care

As we know, healthcare equity is not globally experienced. In places like the UK, Canada, Australia, Sweden, Norway, and Denmark, there are established health and social care systems in place to support

Disabled people and these are free. We are not saying free healthcare is the answer, because we know ableism lurks within the healthcare system.

Whatever the country, the medical model of Disability is there, rooted in these systems, leading Disabled people to seek private medical care options which can be costly, and with the additional expense of living as a Disabled person, it is not always doable. To be a Disabled person living in a country where there is access to free healthcare, even when at times it fails us, is still a privilege many Disabled people do not have.

The World Health Organization reports that 80% of Disabled people globally reside in low- or middle-income countries, where healthcare resources are limited (United Nations Office for Disaster Risk Reduction, 2023).

For those Disabled people residing in these countries this can mean:

- **inaccessible barriers** – healthcare facilities which are not physically accessible

- **financial barriers** – due to poverty and lack of readily available financial support, Disabled people are often unable to afford treatment, assistive technology, medications, rehabilitation, or therapies

- **stigma and discrimination** – cultural beliefs and social stigma can lead to neglect or exclusion for Disabled people in healthcare and within their communities, creating a sense of shame

- **inadequate legal frameworks** – without adequate legal

framework and enforcement of these, Disabled people are more open to discrimination within health and social care

- **transportation barriers** – in countries where public transport is inaccessible, it creates barriers for Disabled people who rely on this to attend appointments.

For those 80% of Disabled people globally, this means barriers to receiving diagnosis, medication, assistive technology, therapy, and rehabilitation – treatment which for many can be life or death.

The World Health Organization (2022) also reports that Disabled people are more likely to experience premature death due to unmet health needs, barriers to healthcare access, and systemic discrimination. Further research by the Centers for Disease Control and Prevention (Okoro *et al.*, 2018) indicates that Disabled people are less likely to receive preventive healthcare, leading to higher rates of chronic illness and avoidable complications. Not having access to healthcare is literally costing Disabled people their lives.

The National Institutes of Health (2023) has officially designated Disabled people as a population facing significant health disparities, reinforcing the urgent need for inclusive laws and equitable health and social care services for Disabled people. Organisations like the World Health Organization and the United Nations work to try to bridge these disparities, but progress is slow and the gap is still wider than we would hope it to be.

Medical capitalism

We live in a capitalist society where private healthcare dominates the market across many countries, creating financial barriers for Disabled people. For example:

- **US:** Private healthcare is the primary system, with government-funded programmes such as Medicare and Medicaid supporting specific groups (Smith, 2023).

- **India:** Public healthcare is underfunded, leading many to rely on private healthcare for quality treatment (Patel, 2022).

- **China:** Private healthcare dominates, with increasing privatisation in hospitals and medical services (Wang & Li, 2021).

- **South Africa:** Private healthcare tends to provide a much better service, but only for those who can afford it (Moyo, 2020).

If we look more closely at the US, although there are legal protections in place to protect Disabled people in healthcare, such as the Americans with Disabilities Act and Section 504 of the Rehabilitation Act, there are still discriminatory practices which restrict Disabled people's ability to receive appropriate care.

Studies have shown that some healthcare providers harbour biases, consciously or unconsciously, leading to substandard care or outright refusal of services to Disabled patients. Research indicates that physicians may express reluctance to treat Disabled patients, citing inadequate facilities or training. A study published in *Health Affairs* found that only 56.5% of physicians strongly agreed that they welcomed patients with Disabilities into their practices, with some expressing a lack of knowledge about providing accommodations and adversarial attitudes towards the Americans with Disabilities Act (Iezzoni *et al.*, 2021).

Additionally, focus groups set up by researchers from Northwestern University Feinberg School of Medicine revealed that some physicians admitted to making strategic choices to deny care to people with

Disabilities, using statements such as, 'I am not taking new patients' or, 'I do not take your insurance' (Lagu *et al.*, 2022). If you are a Disabled person in the US, this means that even if you do have the insurance or the money to pay for private healthcare, you could automatically be denied an appointment simply because you are Disabled.

Disabled people are more likely to be unemployed and living in poverty; in fact, 21.6% of Disabled people in the US were considered poor under the US Census Bureau's Supplemental Poverty Measure, compared to just over 10% of those without Disabilities (Fox, 2020). We, as Disabled people, are often not able to afford medication, assistive technology, or access to health or social care services. If you have to choose between paying insurance or keeping a roof over your head, your healthcare becomes a privilege.

Intersectionality and health and social care

Remember that other systems of oppression, such as racism, will intersect to further compound Disabled individuals and groups with health and social care settings.

In 2022, the uninsured rates for Hispanic and Black adults were 18.7% and 10.9%, respectively, compared to 6.5% for white adults. The following year, in 2023, the uninsured rates slightly decreased to 17.9% for Hispanic adults and 9.7% for Black adults, while the rate for white adults remained steady at 6.5% (Ndugga *et al.*, 2022, 2023).

Meanwhile, in the UK, research shows that ethnic minority groups experienced health inequalities, with some groups more likely to report poorer health and less favourable experiences with healthcare services compared to white groups (Raleigh & Holmes, 2021).

Disabled women also experience additional barriers, affecting how they engage with and experience health and social care. They often face additional bias, assumptions, and, at times, restrictions when trying to access services such as reproductive healthcare diagnoses. For example, ADHD can manifest differently in women, often presenting as inattentiveness rather than hyperactivity. This can lead to misdiagnosis or delays in diagnosis, as traditional diagnostic criteria may not fully capture the female experience of ADHD (Psych Central, 2022). When we add the layer of ethnicity and race to this, things become even more oppressive.

> 66 For years, I thought my struggles were just a by-product of my cross-cultural background – until I was diagnosed with ADHD after my second child was born. Even after that, I felt that ADHD alone didn't fully explain my existential struggles, because the traits within the label covered a 'larger than life' boy experience. As an Asian woman who had long ago learned to wind it back in, I set off to understand our neurodivergent women experience, which led me to finally being assessed for autism.
>
> I was denied the diagnosis three times. They were looking for an autistic white boy in me. They were never going to find him. I pushed back.
>
> Two British women psychologists had assessed me and I challenged their decision, sending research from biology to lived experience. But the reality is, I'm AuDHD, not just autistic. No existing rating scales capture the lived experience of AuDHD women, let alone one from a South East Asian background.
>
> And worse, I had internalised so many societal expectations that I was always carefully putting one foot ahead of the other to 'get it right'. The masks were deeply set in.

While being on ADHD medication, I forgot what it was like to have some of my ADHD struggles. My autistic traits came to the fore. And there were things I couldn't mask, like my extreme literal thinking, which made me seem 'too blunt' or 'slow on the uptake' (from autistic inertia), or my social anxiety, which left me too afraid to say hello in unfamiliar spaces.

By my fourth meeting with my assessors, I was exhausted. Whether they gave me a diagnosis or not, I knew who I was. Seven months after my first assessment, I was finally diagnosed. I cried, not just from relief, but because they told me they had read everything I sent. They re-examined my case, recognised my masking, consulted more clinicians, and even started support groups to help others understand the intersection of ADHD and autism. Too many AuDHD women still face cognitive dissonance, dismissed by male-centric diagnostic criteria. And for those of us with additional intersectional identities, where struggles were hidden or manifested in different ways? We're left unrecognised. Unsupported. Still fighting to be seen. 〞

– Dr Samantha Hiew, Founder of ADHD Girls

ADHD is often underdiagnosed in females, including Black women, due to differences in presentation (Kuehn, 2010). But it is not just when seeking a diagnosis that Disabled Black women experience compounded disadvantage. They also experience the following:

- **Medical discrimination and bias:** Healthcare providers often harbour biases against Black women, and these can be amplified when combined with a Disability. This can result in misdiagnoses, delayed diagnoses, or outright denial of care (BMC Health Services Research, 2021).

- **Higher mortality rates:** Black Disabled women experience higher mortality rates due to lack of access to timely and adequate healthcare services. This is especially pronounced in conditions that require ongoing management or urgent care (Chowdhury *et al.*, 2020).

- **Underrepresentation in medical research:** Black Disabled women are significantly underrepresented in clinical trials and medical research studies. This results in treatments that may not account for the unique needs of this group. Consequently, healthcare solutions tend to be less effective for them (Le *et al.*, 2022).

Unlearning ableism in healthcare means also unlearning sexism, racism, classism, homophobia, transphobia, biphobia, and other systems of oppression.

Disability and mental health

Disabled adults experience frequent mental health distress 4.6 times more often than non-Disabled adults (Cree *et al.*, 2020). In research by Wang *et al.* (2024), Disabled people reported that healthcare providers often held misplaced assumptions about their mental health needs, lacked adequate knowledge about Disability, and sometimes ignored or stereotyped their experiences.

Internalised ableism is often excluded from the mental health conversation and, as we know, internalised ableism is when a Disabled person internalises the ableism they experience, which then can create psychological harm, impacting a person's mental health.

But often, mental health professionals don't seem to understand internalised ableism and instead they take a different approach:

- **They pathologise Disability:** Instead of addressing ableism, some healthcare professionals treat Disability as the problem. 'Oh, you are upset because you can't see, can't walk, can't….' Fill in the blank. They fail to address or understand how ableism negatively impacts mental health. We are not saying that people don't experience loss when they acquire Disability, because they do. Someone acquiring Disability later in life may go through a state of mourning for who they were, or they might experience a sense of loss for what could have been, had they known sooner. But failing to account for ableism and how it impacts a Disabled person is ignoring its emotional toll on a person.

- **They don't provide Disability-affirming therapy:** A lot of healthcare professionals prioritise and encourage patients to achieve 'normalcy' rather than embracing who they are, Disability and all, completely neglecting Disability-affirming care. Disability-affirming care focuses on encouraging people to recognise that it is not their Disability that is the problem, but rather ableism, inaccessibility, and social stigma. This type of care focuses on self-acceptance and empowering a Disabled person, not trying to get them to conform to non-Disabled standards set by a society not designed for them.

- **They use overcoming narratives:** Some therapists are known to use methods which can only be described as toxic positivity. 'You can do anything if you try harder' is a mindset that ignores the limitations a person might have, no matter how much trying they do. This way of treating Disabled people equates our healing to overcoming our Disability – and trust us, if we could overcome Disability by thinking it, we would – and because we cannot overcome it, we must not be trying hard enough, and that is a personal failure on us.

When the impact ableism and internalised ableism has on a Disabled person is not acknowledged, there is a failure to provide adequate mental health services. Trust us, we have been in enough healthcare professionals' offices literally screaming and crying about how ableism has made us feel, only to be ignored and told we need to try harder to get on with it.

Social care

Social care for Disabled people is meant to be centred around helping Disabled people achieve independence, ensuring well-being, dignity, autonomy, and of course, ensuring that Disabled people are included across society. It should provide access to daily assistance if required, healthcare, and mental health services. All sounds pretty straightforward, right?

We want Disabled people to be included, supported, and free of barriers, don't we?

But access to social care services for Disabled people is not easy. As in healthcare and all other systems within society, ableism has taken root and creates barriers for Disabled service users. Let's take a look at these.

Limited funding/resources

As many social care services for Disabled people are underfunded, this can lead to longer waiting lists, insufficient support, and reduced services. Budget cuts can make it harder for Disabled people to access these essential services. A survey revealed that four in five Disabled people faced cuts in care packages or increased charges during the pandemic, with providers reporting that council fee rates were not keeping pace with costs (Community Care, 2021). For many Disabled people, such cuts to funding mean being left for hours alone, unable to get themselves to the bathroom or make meals.

Inaccessibility

We know we use this word a lot, but accessibility encompasses so many different things! For Disabled people, accessing social care can be difficult due to physical barriers, such as buildings not having access, and communication barriers, where patients do not get sign interpreters or information in appropriate alternative formats such as easy read material, braille, or large font. A 2022 study published in *Health Affairs* identified numerous physical, communication, and structural obstacles that impede access to care for people with Disabilities (Iezzoni *et al.*, 2021). The study also revealed that some physicians, overwhelmed by the need to accommodate these patients, have discharged them from their practices.

Lack of training and workforce shortages

A lot of people working within the social care setting have limited exposure to diverse Disabilities or can lack the necessary training required to support Disabled service users. There is also a workforce shortage of staff, resulting in issues with Disabled people not receiving consistent care or not getting the right level of care. A report by Skills for Care (2022) identified that there were 165,000 vacant care roles in England, which impacted service provision.

Complex applications and eligibility criteria

Many Disabled people struggle with the complex application processes that they regularly face when it comes to social care services. These applications often require extensive documentation and medical proof. Strict eligibility assessments can often disqualify Disabled people, due to their rigid criteria or staff who have little awareness when making assessments. An example of this is the UK welfare benefit, Personal Independence Payment (PIP). This is designed to help individuals with long-term physical, mental health conditions or Disabilities, providing financial support to cover costs related to daily living and mobility difficulties. However, over the past decade, the success rate for PIP appeals has significantly increased, raising concerns about the application and decision-making process and how many people are being turned down on their initial application (Pring, 2019).

Cost of social care

In many countries, social care is not funded or not fully funded. This means Disabled people must pay for some or all of their care. As we are learning in this book though, access to these services is a privilege which many Disabled people cannot afford. In the US, for example, the cost of long-term care can be overwhelming, as many Disabled people must either pay out-of-pocket or rely on limited insurance coverage. A study from the National Health Interview Survey (2020) found that over 20% of Disabled people spend a significant portion of their income on medical and care-related expenses. Moreover, many states have strict eligibility criteria for Medicaid, which provides assistance for long-term care, leaving Disabled individuals without adequate financial support for necessary services.

Lack of person-centred care

Within social care services there tends to be the same rigid, one-size-fits-all approach, which overlooks a Disabled individual, their needs, preferences, and autonomy. This can lead to professionals making decisions about care plans without centring the patient first and leading to a loss of their independence. A report by *The Guardian* in January 2025 highlighted that systemic failures and ingrained prejudices have led to significant challenges for Disabled adults, including isolation and lack of support. The report emphasised that nearly 50% of care spending supports Disabled adults of working age, with the majority being for those with learning Disabilities. It also noted that Disabled individuals often find themselves isolated, with limited community access, causing stress and anxiety (Harris, 2025).

It's time to unlearn ableism in health and social care

Now unless you work in health and social care, you're probably wondering what this has got to do with you and how you can change this. Well, if you are a healthcare professional, therapist, doctor, care worker, support worker, nurse, and so on, we hope this next part of the chapter will help you become an anti-ableist practitioner! If you are not, we hope you read on anyway, as lots of this learning is transferable!

Unlearning ableism in health and social care starts with understanding that yes, the medical model of Disability has had its place, but we need to shift to a social model lens.

Shifting to a social model lens

Health and social care workers need to see people as individuals. A textbook won't tell you how people experience Disability. A textbook medical answer will not tell you how a person's internalised ableism impacts their mental health, how their race and ethnicity also impact this. It will not tell you beyond a generic textbook response. Listen to your patients. Recognise the ableism and inaccessibility that we deal with daily, look at long-term treatment plans, don't just try to fix us. By looking at Disability through the lens of the social model, rather than the medical model, you can begin to understand the complexities of what it means to be a Disabled person, because it is not just our conditions that disable us; it is ableism, it is inaccessibility, it is discrimination that take their toll on us.

Education and awareness

If you're not aware, you cannot hope to unlearn ableism. Healthcare professionals need a better understanding of what ableism is and how it operates in healthcare settings. They also need to be aware of how they contribute to it. Be sure to attend any training, seminars, or workshops that are focused on Disability, anti-ableism, and diversity in healthcare. It's okay to say you do not know, but it's not okay to let yourself be guided by a textbook response which you yourself don't truly understand. The saying, 'You only know what you don't know', should be embraced by healthcare professionals when it comes to ableism.

Challenge your inner ableism

In order to challenge your inner ableism, you need to be open to self-reflection – being aware of your own bias, prejudice, and assumptions that you have or make about Disabled patients. You might think before meeting a blind person that they won't be able to see, when we know blindness is a spectrum and the person potentially has some sight. Avoid making generalisations or imposing stereotypes about who fits what category, 'Well, this young girl is verbal so she can't possibly be autistic.' These kinds of generalisations only reinforce ableist stereotypes.

Consider your language

We get it, you work in healthcare, you probably joined to help or make people feel better – an incredibly beautiful thing to want to do for others. We know you want to help ease our suffering when we are sore, to help fix us where you can, but we need you to understand that we aren't always suffering from our Disability. Doctors have asked us if we are still suffering from [insert Disability here]. We are not all suffering, not all wheelchair users are wheelchair bound, not all Disability is as black and white as you might believe. Be mindful of your language, be inclusive, don't assume, and ask us how we want to self-identify. You calling us a 'person with Disability' when we have asked to be called a 'Disabled person' is just rude.

Focus on person-centred care

Let us have control over our own care! We need to have autonomy when it comes to making decisions about how we want to be treated. You making decisions about us without consulting us undermines us and literally strips us of our autonomy. Be flexible when working with patients, ask about their access needs and preferred way of communicating, and be sure to provide information in accessible formats if a patient has requests. We know that you have probably spent a long time in your career in healthcare, but we have spent years living with our Disabilities, so respect that you won't always have the answer and that is okay, that's why you need to involve us – the Disabled patients – in the conversation.

View Disability through an intersectional lens

Health and social care workers need to understand that a person's experience of Disability doesn't exist in a vacuum; it's shaped by so many other factors. Just as a textbook won't tell you how someone is experiencing Disability, it also won't show you how their race, gender, sexuality, or class is impacting the care they receive. An intersectional lens recognises that it's not about Disability in isolation; it's about how all these aspects of a person's identity interact, shaping their experience of healthcare. Ask Disabled people who are also part of marginalised communities – whether that's Black, LGBTQIA+ – what we need. Recognise how systemic oppression, ableism, racism, sexism, and classism are at play in our healthcare experiences.

Only by looking through an intersectional lens will you begin to understand the layers of oppression that can impact our health and well-being. It's not just about treating us; it's about understanding the complex web of barriers that shape our experiences. These barriers are not just physical, but deeply rooted in society's prejudices – and your own biases too.

66 As a Disabled therapist working in healthcare for over 20 years, I've seen and felt the impact of ableism. For a while now, I've been passionately raising awareness about ableism and internalised ableism in my health organisation. It is important not just to talk about ableism within our Disability communities, but to get this message out to all levels of an organisation. I urge you to have ableism as part of the vocabulary in healthcare settings. Bring it to the attention of your senior leadership teams and governing boards, incorporate it in team meetings.

When discussing clinical practices, have open conversations on whether the practice is Disability affirming or is actually ableist. For many of us in healthcare, the notion of unlearning ableism is a journey. It can be uncomfortable to reflect on and acknowledge that some of the healthcare practices we've done for many years could be ableist. But I encourage you to lean into the uncomfortable, listen to the stories, and then change the narrative. Discomfort and deep reflection can be powerful catalysts for positive change. Embrace it, listen to your Disabled patients – and to your Disabled staff too – and work together to rewrite the narrative.

Disabled staff and patients bring invaluable lived experience and offer perspectives that are crucial in delivering excellent healthcare. Always make sure Disabled people are part of the conversation – don't other us. To non-Disabled healthcare staff, we need you, we need allies who are committed to this agenda. My advice to Disabled healthcare staff is to come together in your organisation, whether you use the word Disabled or not. While your diagnoses may differ, what you will find is that you all encounter ableism on a regular basis, and can be united in wanting to break down the many barriers you face as Disabled healthcare staff and as patients in the healthcare system.

You are stronger together if you have these bigger, wider strategic conversations on tackling ableism in health. I finish with the words from someone who has become a great non-Disabled ally to me and the Disability community in health, 'Get your sledgehammers out.' This is a call to action! "

– Mary Lavender, autistic speech and language therapist and Disability advocate

We are not just people to be fixed or managed; we are people with multifaceted identities who deserve care that acknowledges and respects all of who we are.

The experiences of Disabled people in health and social care cannot be shared in one chapter, one book, or by one person. There are millions of stories of people who are being failed, let down, and not being provided with access to a fundamental human right, health.

To end this chapter, we leave this final message for healthcare professionals. We know you put a lot of time, dedication, and energy into your profession. We know how underappreciated healthcare professionals can be, but we see you and we really do appreciate you. But please, see us, hear us, and learn from us. When communicating with us, please don't use fancy language, jargon, or complicated explanations. Make information accessible and, for the love of inclusion, help us build healthcare literacy.

CHAPTER 14

Unlearning Ableism: Entrepreneurs and Economics

> **Abba sings about money and how it is a rich man's world.**
> **It's not a Disabled one though.**

We cannot possibly examine life as a Disabled person, waging battles against an ableist world, without discussing the financial implications of being Disabled – and goodness, it's expensive out here!

From point A to point Z in following each piece of money that comes in and out of our pockets, from purchasing and spending power, to the additional financial implications of – heaven forbid – trying to make money ourselves away from the barriers of traditional employment, yup, you've guessed it, ableism continues to get in our way.

Disability spending power

Let's start by looking at purchasing and spending power. How easy is it for Disabled people to be able to actually spend the money we have? Well, although we are 17% of the global population, do not be fooled into thinking that it would be logical for organisations to ensure that their services and products are open and available to their Disabled consumers – pfft, how silly that would be?!

The World Health Organization (2022) estimates that the more than 1.3 billion Disabled people around the world, alongside their friends and family, have a spending power of $13 trillion. To put that into numbers, one trillion is one million-million-million, so times that again by 13. And in the UK, the spending power of Disabled people is known as the Purple Pound, and estimated to be upwards of £274 billion every single year (Purple, n.d). In the US, this is known as the Purple Dollar and the American Institutes for Research (Yin *et al.*, 2018) reports that Disabled people in the US have a disposable income of approximately $490 billion.

That's a lot of dollars!

And are we making use of it? Of course not! Research shows that the spending power of Disabled people is not being utilised:

- Seventy-three per cent of Disabled shoppers shopping online say they have experienced barriers on more than a quarter of the websites that they have visited (Purple, n.d).

- Pure-play e-commerce retailers in the US are estimated to lose over $6.9 billion annually due to non-compliance with accessibility standards (Gevorkian, 2024).

- Seventy-two per cent of Disabled consumers have abandoned a purchase because of accessibility issues on websites or apps (Jenkins, 2024).

- Businesses in the UK lose approximately £2 billion every single month by ignoring the needs of Disabled people (Purple, n.d.).

But why aren't we utilising the spending power of Disabled people?

It's our friend ableism yet again, creating barriers for Disabled people in being able to access the products and services that we want and need or not even having the choice of or access to inclusive and accessible products and services.

These barriers include: inaccessible built environments and transport links, making in-person shopping impossible; inaccessible digital consumer platforms, making online shopping impossible; in accessibilities in banking and building societies, making management of and access to finances difficult. Add to this list poor consumer experiences, inaccessible price points, and a lack of adaptive or accessible products.

By dismantling these ableism barriers for Disabled people, we reap the benefits not only socially but also economically. Disabled people, as the largest minority group in the world, are one of the largest consumer market segments. A study conducted by Accenture, in partnership with Disability:IN and the American Association of People with Disabilities (2018), found that profit margins were 30% higher and net income was 200% higher for companies invested in hiring employees who were Disabled, because they were able to better meet the needs of their consumers.

Part 1: How can we remove ableism from our economics?

Let's explore barriers for Disabled consumers, and some ways of removing them and allowing for the utilisation of our spending power:

- **Accessibility barriers, both physically and digitally:** If Disabled people can't access goods and services, how on earth are we supposed to make a purchase? There must be greater thought given to the environments that are built, creating engagement not preventing it, and breaking down barriers for Disabled people to enable us to participate, and enjoy being consumers.

- **Awareness and education:** The inherent lack of knowledge of the existence, size, and significance of Disability spending power means that focus on the barriers and remedial action required is not where it should be. Better awareness and education will address knowledge gaps and utilise potential to cause astronomical economic shifts.

- **Marketing and advertising:** Truly inclusive and accessible marketing and advertising to Disabled consumers will improve choice and opportunity.

- **Stigma and bias:** Breaking down outdated and incorrect attitudes will prevent automatic exclusion in various consumer markets, affecting how products and services are designed and marketed.

- **Internal and external representation:** Current representation in marketing and within company roles leads to inherent failures for Disabled people across design, manufacture, and delivery, and prevents due attention being paid to needs, accessibility, and preference. There should be: nothing about us without us.

- **Disability employment:** This encompasses everything we have discussed in our employment chapter again, again, and again!

- **Policy, law and regulation:** A lack of incentives, basic requirements of accessibility, and undue care and focus for the movement of goods and services for Disabled people lead to missed opportunities in tapping into the Disability market.

- **Macro and micro economic factors:** Unemployment, healthcare, security, and access to opportunity are all factors in how and why we choose to spend our money.

- **Qualitative and quantitative data captures:** There is still a significant lack of comprehensive data on the purchasing powers, behaviours, and preferences of Disabled people needed to create effective strategies and break down biases.

To better utilise Disability spending power, it is essential for businesses, organisations, regulatory bodies, and governments to recognise the value of inclusivity, invest in accessibility, and develop strategies that resonate and are accessible to all Disabled people.

The Disability Price Tag

Although we've got the spending power, please don't be fooled into imagining that Disabled people are simply trundling around with money heaving out of our pockets practically begging someone to take it from us. Actually, it's quite the opposite. To be a Disabled person strips us of financial privilege the majority of the time.

The World Bank estimates that 20% of the world's poorest people identify as Disabled (United Nations Department of Economic and Social Affairs, n.d.), while Disability Rights UK (2022b) states that nearly half of the people living in poverty in the UK in 2021–2022 were Disabled. And the United Nations Development Programme (n.d.) reports that 80% of Disabled people live in developing countries, which often correlates with lower income levels. In the most horrific of languages, we are known globally as 'The Bottom Billion'.

Poverty and Disability go hand-in-hand, reinforcing one another and creating a cycle of shortage and deprivation, where it seems impossible to break free.

Because of our identity, for the majority of us our destiny to live below the average standard of living is set, not only because of the systemic lack of opportunities for participation and progress across health, education, transportation, information, and services, that we have already discussed throughout this book, but also because of the costs associated with being a Disabled person – the Disability Price Tag.

The Disability Price Tag refers to the additional costs that Disabled people face as a direct consequence of their Disability or health condition. These can be direct or indirect costs. Direct costs include the expenses which directly relate to the Disability; indirect costs are things such as loss of income or lack of opportunities or progressions as a consequence of ableism.

The Scope Disability Price Tag report (2024) found that in the UK 'on average, Disabled households need an additional £1,010 a month to have the same standard of living as non-Disabled households, and the extra cost of Disability is equivalent to 67% of household income after housing costs'. And according to the National Disability Institute (2020), a household with an adult with a Disability in the US 'needs approximately 28% more income to maintain the same standard of living as a household without a Disability, which translates to an extra $17,690 per year at the median income level'.

To put it oh so eloquently and simply: it's bloody expensive to be Disabled! Not only do we have to deal with the physical and mental battles of being Disabled, we've got to struggle financially as well.

Examples of these costs include adapted equipment, dressings and covers, transport for medical appointments, interpreters, adaptive and assistive technology, care providers, housing modifications, higher utility bills such as heating, and higher insurance rates. In other words, costs we wouldn't have to bear if it weren't for our health. Now this all sounds very medical model, doesn't it? Well, you'd be right: because of our Disability we are having to pay the consequences; as Disabled people we should just suck it up, expect it, and allow for it.

But therein lies the problem. Due to the lack of choices of adapted equipment, prices are higher than non-adapted equipment. Because of the lack of mainstream education for Disability service providers, such as sign language interpreters and transcribers, services remain specialised and priced high. Because of medical biases, costs of insurance and necessary medical equipment are high. Because of inaccessibilities in the built environment, and within transport networks, accessible transport costs are higher.

So yes, we have to pay for things that non-Disabled people don't, but the enormous costs of these goods and services are so high, how are we supposed to stand an economic chance? These additional costs we have to face are the living demonstration of why a shift to the social model of Disability is so necessary, and a key component of unlearning ableism: opening up choice, opportunity, and consumerism for all.

Part 2: How can we remove ableism from our economics?

Let's consider the creation of choice, policies, support systems, and inclusive consumer practices that lessen the financial burdens faced by Disabled people. We are faced with oligopolies and monopolies, where what we need are competitive market structures, just like everybody else.

Disabled entrepreneurialism

According to Cambridge Dictionary (n.d.a), an entrepreneur is someone who 'starts their own business, especially when it involves seeing new opportunities and new ideas'.

We've talked about employment, recruitment, and the end-to-end barriers Disabled people face in the workplace, but there's another 'workplace' we have not discussed. Entrepreneurs – our Disabled entrepreneurs designing, redesigning, re-imagining, and paving a way forward that is more accessible, inclusive, and choice driven.

Disabled people over-index on attributes such as resilience, creativity, empathy, determination, and the ability to think outside the box, all attributes sought by entrepreneurs. And given the barriers we face in employment markets, naturally a lot of Disabled people divert to working for themselves.

But it isn't all sunshine and roses. Yes, we are trailblazing, but swimming with all the currents against us.

Data captured by Access2Funding highlights a troubling and significant gap in the investment opportunities available to businesses owned and led by Disabled people. Despite making up over 17% of the global population, Disabled people currently hold just 0.1% of the total investment share. According to a survey of Disabled entrepreneurs, more than 97% felt there was a lack of visibility for their businesses, while 75.6% believed they did not have equal access to the same opportunities and resources as their non-Disabled counterparts. Of the remaining 24.4%, 19.5% felt they only sometimes had equal opportunity and access to resources. Furthermore, 83.7% of respondents reported that investment opportunities for Disabled entrepreneurs were inconsistent in terms of equity.

Entrepreneurs with Disabilities face multiple, systemic barriers throughout the investment process, including accessibility challenges, limited participation opportunities, ableism, inaccessible applications and systems, misconceptions about risk management, and a general lack of awareness about the capabilities of Disabled individuals.

Among those who were unable to secure capital, 48.4% cited a lack of support and advice tailored to Disabled entrepreneurs, 45.2% believed they lacked the same access to investors as non-Disabled entrepreneurs, and 41.9% pointed to inadequate resources. Another 32.3% couldn't find relevant information for Disabled entrepreneurs, while 29% felt that investors prioritised other concerns over those of Disabled entrepreneurs. Over 32% of respondents felt that a combination of these factors led to their inability to secure funding.

Alarmingly, only 10.3% of Disabled entrepreneurs believed they were treated equally to their non-Disabled peers when it came to investment opportunities (Access2Funding, 2023).

These statistics about life as a Disabled entrepreneur, trying to compete, makes the mind boggle. Breaking down barriers for Disabled entrepreneurs involves addressing a variety of systemic, social, and economic Disability barriers that are actively contributing to ableism within our society.

Part 3: How can we remove ableism from our economics?

So let's now look at the utilisation of Disabled entrepreneurialism, and how that can increase.

- Open funding to all, creating inclusive investment systems, developing accessible venture capital flows and programmes.

- Improve access to education and knowledge for Disabled people; open training and development opportunities with fully accessible resources.

- Open mentorship, networking, and allyship opportunities to provide guidance and support to Disabled founders. Build networks and promote connections.

- Advocate for policy and regulatory changes that promote inclusion and remove barriers for Disabled founders, and encourage growth through incentives, improved representation, and opportunities for participation.

- Raise public and business awareness of the talent and potential of Disabled people, breaking down biases and stereotypes, inspiring and demonstrating the validity of Disabled power.

- Remove inaccessible barriers across workplaces, the built environment, digital spaces, platforms, and businesses to improve Disability involvement and open opportunity.

- Operate with inclusive practices and diverse workplaces and workforces to foster open, honest, and inclusive sustainable environments.

We think you'll agree, all of these sound very much like unlearning ableism to us!

Why is it so important to support Disabled entrepreneurs?

Supporting Disabled entrepreneurs will increase spending power by driving income, opening choice, and improving the accessibility of existing and entering markets. Disabled entrepreneurs bring unique perspectives, innovative solutions, and new opportunities, and ultimately drive economic growth, helping to dismantle ableism barriers from the inside out. We provide:

- creativity, market gap identification, and innovative inclusive solutions

- creation of market access and utilisation of spending power

- valuable assets such as problem solving, determination, diverse perspective, and resilience to micro- and macro-economic challenges

- individual and community economic empowerment

- increase in the social impact of accessibility, intersectionality, and inclusion

- economic growth through business contribution, job creation, and consumer power

- increased Disability visibility and representation.

Breaking down the systemic ableism barriers for Disabled entrepreneurs is not only a matter of social justice but also an essential step towards creating economic empowerment, innovation, and inclusivity. By creating an environment that supports and nurtures Disabled entrepreneurs, as a society we can unlock greater potential to enrich our society as a whole.

> " Four years ago, my company, Clu, made it to the final round of one of Europe's top investment pitch competitions – a game-changing moment for any startup. But when I arrived, I faced a

flight of stairs and no alternative access. The organisers could do nothing and told me to apply again next year. That moment crystallised a brutal reality: Disabled entrepreneurs don't just navigate the challenges of building a business; we battle systemic exclusion at every stage. Disabled founders own one in four small and medium sized enterprises in the UK, yet we are 400 times less likely to secure investment than our non-Disabled peers. That's not just unjust – it's an economic failure, leaving almost £1 billion in returns on the table each year. Through Access2Funding, we exposed the systemic inaccessibility of the UK's venture ecosystem. The research confirmed what we already knew – Disabled entrepreneurs have the same ambitions but are consistently blocked from accessing networks, capital, and opportunities. Clu is now a seed-stage company, but I'm too aware I'm one of very few who've made it this far. Too few of us break through, despite having everything it takes. We over-index in the very traits that define the world's most successful founders: creativity, resilience, determination, and problem-solving. It's no coincidence that history proves that many of the greatest innovators have been Disabled or neurodiverse – our make-up is exceptional, which is why despite these barriers, we already contribute 8% of GDP in the UK. Imagine the contribution we could make with the system on our side. 🙶

– Joseph Williams, CEO, Clu

Why do we need to unlearn ableism in our economic markets?

Research from Concern Worldwide (2023) explains the 'Cycle of Poverty' is a reinforcing cycle of deprivation that traps people in poverty across generations, also known as the 'Poverty Trap'.

Going back to Chapter 5 on the history of Disability, the historical inherent nature of society to act with a medical model approach has entrenched ableism within our economical patterns, limiting the financial and economic freedom of Disabled people, trapping us within the constraints of ableism.

We are stuck chasing our tails, going round and round in a loop of limited discretionary spending, and above average non-discretionary spending, prevented from entering employment but then faced with additional barriers when we try to go it alone. This is the medical model signalling to us loud and clear that we are the problem, the cost, the burden.

To break down economic Disability barriers and to create equity of financial opportunity is to break this cycle and create a knock-on effect of positive change across all aspects of a person's life – employment, participation, survival, and thriving – for after all, money really does make the world go round.

Removing ableism from economics not only benefits Disabled people but also society as a whole. We must shift the burden of responsibility away from Disabled people and all take responsibility to unlock their untapped potential.

> 66 Disability and entrepreneurship are often perceived as unrelated, but in truth, they are deeply intertwined. Living with a Disability presents unique barriers that can make traditional employment challenging – if not entirely inaccessible – due to workplace inaccessibility, employer biases, and rigid job structures. For many Disabled individuals, entrepreneurship isn't just an option; it's a necessity. However, starting and sustaining a business as a Disabled entrepreneur comes with

its own set of challenges. One of the biggest hurdles is access to finance, as many financial institutions and investors wrongly perceive Disabled entrepreneurs as high risk. Additionally, societal biases can make it harder to gain credibility, secure funding, and establish meaningful business networks. Yet, with the right approach, these barriers can be overcome. I am living proof that success is possible. My strategy has always been to develop a strong business model with a clear niche market, and then dominate that space. For example, I founded one of the first digital marketing agencies in the Midlands and launched the UK's first free web-hosting service. Continuous self-development has also been key. Every year, I challenge myself to learn something new. For example, a few years ago, I learned how to trade, and today, it provides me with an additional income stream. Adaptability is crucial – challenges and setbacks will happen, but they should be viewed as stepping stones, not roadblocks. Entrepreneurship offers independence, flexibility, and the opportunity to build inclusive workplaces. Disability and entrepreneurship are not opposites; together, they are catalysts for innovation and change. 99

– Mark Esho MBE

CHAPTER 15

Unlearning Ableism: Allyship Is More than a Word...

Reading one book won't suddenly make you the most super-duper, anti-ableist ally ever! Likewise, saying you support Disabled people doesn't suddenly win you a medal of inclusion. Allyship is so much more than someone claiming to be an ally.

We have come to the end – well, the last chapter anyway – and you are on your merry way to unlearning ableism, but what happens after you read this book? How do you put all you have learned into practice? How do you bring these lessons out into society?

Be proactive, not reactive

Unlearning ableism through action, not being passive standers-by, being proactive, not reactive, acting with anticipatory duty, and being forward-thinking, not stagnant. We have to take charge of our own destiny; if we do nothing, we do not move forward. We cannot be submissive to the ableism that blankets us all – we must act!

This is your call to action. Allies assemble! March onwards! Let's take the bull by the horns.

Ninety-five per cent of Disabled people have experienced ableism – that's 1,235,000,000 Disabled people; 46.6% of Disabled people experience ableism at least once a week – that's 605,800,000 people (Disabled by Society, 2024). Why? Because we are failing to take action.

Before we dive in, let's first understand what we mean by ally.

What does it mean to be an ally?

An ally is someone who actively supports and stands up for the rights and interests of a marginalised or disadvantaged group, even if they do not belong to that group themselves. It's about more than just expressing support; it's a heartfelt commitment to understanding, addressing, and taking action.

- **We listen and we learn:** We understand perspectives different from our own; we look within our systems not just on the surface, to be educated and inquisitive with intentional respect.

- **We use our visibility and voice:** We use our privileges and platforms to elevate others to an equal playing field. We share stories, speak out against discrimination, challenge the status quo, and we break down barriers to open the floor for others to always be heard and consulted.

- **We take action:** It isn't about passive support; we are active and dedicated to creating sustainable tangible change. We work in our own spheres of influence to address bias and challenge the behaviors of others through education and recommendation.

- **We acknowledge our privilege:** We recognise the privileges we hold and understand how these have affected our perspectives and actions, contributing to the dynamics of power and oppression. We use this privilege to open spaces and disrupt systems.

- **We are open to criticism and further learning:** As we evolve as a society, so too does the environment around us. Our process of learning is never finished, so we have to be steadfast in our commitments; we have to build trust and demonstrate genuine commitments, and always be willing to learn from our mistakes (which we all make!).

- **We build relationships:** We do not speak on behalf of people, but help create spaces for others to be heard. We engage and understand diversity, intersectionality, and self-expression, never stepping over the boundary of disrespecting the autonomy of a community.

- **We are sustained in our allyship:** Being an ally is not a one-time or short-term thing; we are consistent, engaged, and committed.

Hello again to our favourite and perhaps most crucial word 'active'!

Disabled people are the largest minority group in the world. Despite this, ableism is one of the most under-addressed, under-discussed, and underrepresented conversations in society. Society is failing to unlearn its inherent ableism. Every day, millions of Disabled people face macro- and microaggressions, encounter inaccessible barriers, are excluded, overlooked, treated as a burden, and seen as a problem to be fixed. As a result, Disabled people are often left to manage internalised ableism in this ableist society. It's a call to action. We have to be on a mission to change this. We can no longer sit back and do nothing. Individuals, organisations, governments...we *can* remove the ableism ingrained in cultures, recruitment, products and services, policies, and everything in between. We have to proactively make the uncomfortable comfortable. We have to end this cycle of oppression and create an inclusive society that is accessible, empowers, represents, and provides opportunity and participation for everyone.

> 66 Being a best friend and a carer, although these are similar in thinking, is a complete dichotomy at times. It is being present and an observer at the same time but without becoming overbearing or too aloof. It is encouragement and enthusiasm without limits but also a constantly watchful eye over any minute change in the well-being of the person in front of you. The complexity of the relationship looms in an uncertainty that each incoming phone call may be from a medical facility. It is not a matter of if, but when, the next event may lead to you having to switch roles. The overlap in the two positions is anchored by elephantine proportions of love, but navigating the boundary of when you have to prioritise welfare over 'the fun choice' is forever a challenge – but it is one I would not trade for anything. The people in our lives facing these unsolvable health obstacles daily are often the most extraordinary and that is worth everything. However, convincing those we care for that they are not a burden remains something I have yet to solve. 99

– Heloise Hoare, testimonial carer vs friend

How do you feel about racism? Sexism? Homophobia? Transphobia? Do you feel the same about ableism?

We know that 17% of the world's population identifies as Disabled, and this figure is growing every single year. Only 40 years ago it was estimated that only 10% of the world's population was Disabled. Why? Ageing populations, growing populations, increased exposure, environmental changes, better diagnosis, better life expectancies, better treatments…whatever the reasons may be, as a society we have failed to take action to tackle ableism throughout our history, and look where we are now. Where are we going to be in another 40 years if action does not come now?

Accountability and responsibility

We need to take accountability, identify our previous errors, find our flaws, and take responsibility to end this cycle of oppression. Most of the time, accountability and responsibility are squished together into a single entity, but moving forward we must separate them to create effective progression.

Despite being interlinked in their nature, responsibility and accountability are two separate definable premises, which coupled together are fundamental to ensuring the effective identification and removal of ableism, and improving Disability opportunities and outcomes.

The creation of responsibility and accountability must therefore be a constant and centralised theme of how we can all unlearn ableism, whether that is individually, in organisations, or societal bodies.

Responsibility refers to the duty held by each of us to ensure the execution of positive action both collectively and individually, with the intended mindset of an expected and desired consequence. Through responsibility, there exists the active pursuit of action with intention for the fulfilment of commitment. Effective responsibility creates action for the benefit of Disabled people, improving outcomes and opportunities. Responsibility therefore paves the path for accountability.

Accountability refers not to the dutiful action itself, but draws focus on the consequence of action, the active pursuit by us all to hold ownership of the resulting effects of our actions. Accountability fosters an environment where the effectiveness of action is examined, in its implementation, management, and supporting policies. Effective accountability creates long-term, sustained implementation of Disability equity, inclusion, and accessibility measures as we all learn and develop from our previous actions.

Let's think of an example here

Ted was a project manager in his local community, focused on creating a community garden to promote sustainable living and provide fresh produce for families in need. He was excited about the project and took the lead in organising the efforts. As the project progressed, Ted noticed that some aspects of the garden planning were falling behind schedule. He had delegated tasks to various volunteers, but due to miscommunication and lack of clear instructions, several important deadlines were missed. The garden's opening was pushed back, which disappointed many community members who were looking forward to it. Instead of placing the blame on his volunteers for not meeting deadlines, Ted called a community meeting to address the situation. He openly acknowledged his role in the miscommunication and took full responsibility for the project's setbacks. Ted explained how he could have provided clearer guidance and better support to the volunteers.

Accountability is multifaceted in its benefits, with each of these benefits contributing to the achievement of unlearning ableism:

- Accountability embeds responsibility, ensuring that goals and desired achievements are set, monitored, reassessed, and executed, such as adopting accessibility provisions ameliorating accessible experiences. For example, ensuring accessibility online.

- Accountability is crucial for the promotion of productivity, sustainability of action, and long-term dedication to defined responsibilities. This dedication creates excellence in performance, ensuring that Disability measures imposed are as effective as possible and widespread in their implementation. For example, implementing and regularly updating Disability law.

- Accountability provides context and transparency to responsibilities, and proposes action, assisting in the effective achievement of results. Through the active promotion of the purpose of action, all of us have a greater awareness for the necessity of inclusivity and accessibility. Alongside the motivation for this desired increase, this contextual background encourages greater participation from the community as a whole to the cause of the concern for the lack of accessibility, and diversity is further understood. For example, having better Disability education in schools means that our future generations are more likely to be focused on ableism.

- Accountability sets and maintains expectations for the promotion of success, ameliorating opportunities for participation and engagement for Disabled people.

So as you can now see, accountability and, as a consequence due to their interlinked nature, responsibility are therefore vital in their contribution to our journey in unlearning ableism through action.

Where do we start? And who are we asking to take this accountability and responsibility?

Well, it's all of us. None of us is exempt, whether Disabled or not. Taking action is the responsibility of us all. Just because somebody is Disabled, it does not mean that we automatically know everything there is to know about Disability. Each of our lived experiences is unique to us, and doesn't always shed insight into others' experiences. At point of diagnosis, a beam of light doesn't automatically transfer the entire United Nations Convention of the Rights of Persons with Disabilities into our brains or download some handbook on what we actually need.

We all have to play our part in removing ableism from our society.

We have to reframe our 'deal flow'. With honesty and intention, we highlight our failures and take recommendations to create access, support, and equity. Take our hand; we'll take you through it.

The reframing deal flow

1. **Identify:** Recognise, understand, and acknowledge ableism and Disability.

2. **Challenge:** Question validity, gather evidence, seek alternative perspectives, and reframe your thinking.

3. **Positive affirmation:** Take action, be proactive, instigate the social model, realign key focuses, and celebrate Diversity.

4. **Compassion:** Exercise kindness, understanding, prioritisation, awareness, and care for self and others.

And there we go: allyship in a step-by-step nutshell (well, in partnership with everything else we've said in the entire book), and learning about racism, sexism, homophobia, biphobia, and so on.

But the conversation about accountability and responsibility creating action to unlearn ableism doesn't end there; oh no, there's a whole other wormhole to open and explore.

First of all, and we're saying it loud and clear for those who haven't got it yet. When we say everyone, we mean everyone! Yes, it's the equity of the burden of responsibility. Now, before anyone comes at us for the word burden, we aren't suggesting tackling discrimination as a burden. We have established at this point that unlearning ableism is the provision of human rights and that is definitely not a burden, and if you still think it is this late in the book, we rather fear a lost cause here!

The word burden is used here in line with the 'common phrasing' for reaffirming the duty for accessibility, usability, inclusivity, and equity. These are not 'burdens' but rather the installation and maintenance of legal, ethical, and social responsibilities. Disabled people and access requirements are not to be associated with the word burden, which would imply that the onus of responsibility has been unduly and unfairly placed, inciting negative connotations around Disability.

Now that we have cleared that up, what do we mean by the equity of the burden of responsibility?

In line with the social model of Disability, the improvement of opportunity and outcomes for Disabled people does not fall on Disabled people alone, but also on wider society to provide opportunities and outcomes, regardless of stage, size, category, or sector. Both accountability and responsibility are to be upheld to the utmost degree by those responsible for the production of opportunity and outcomes, either individually or collectively. Currently, there exists an enormous 'disproportionate burden' where Disabled people have been left feeling as if we are steering the unmanned ship on our own, without the allyship we need.

Continuing our narrative of our sailing ship, we flow along the sea nicely into the role of allyship and why it is so vital in our action to unlearn ableism. An ally is also defined as 'an active support for the rights of a minority or marginalised group without being a member of it' (Oxford English Dictionary, n.d.b). See that word active – correct allyship isn't tokenism or stagnant. It should be proactive. Allyship is so important because it involves individuals, particularly those in positions of privilege, actively supporting and advocating for other communities – speaking up, calling out behaviour, amplifying underrepresented and forgotten voices, and taking action to address systemic ableism. By utilising positions of privilege, allies help to create inclusion and equity, rebalancing powers, opening opportunities, and improving outcomes.

Privilege is a word that has the power to spark great debate and great divide. Privilege as a noun is defined as 'an advantage that one person or group of people has over another' (Cambridge Dictionary, n.d.d). Non-Disabled people have privilege over Disabled people (we completely respect and acknowledge intersectionality in this conversation, noting that this statement does not always apply, and recognising the privileges that some Disabled people have over other Disabled people – head to Chapter 4 on intersectionality to learn more!).

In this context, when we speak of privilege we speak of the advantages and benefits that non-Disabled people have over Disabled people: access to opportunities, resources, non-judgemental stereotypes, education, quality of care, expectations... By recognising our own benefits we hold in a system of unbalanced power we can advocate and challenge.

Allyship promotes the equity of opportunity to transform outcome (another rhetoric we ought to touch on). Creating inclusive accessibility, opportunity, and participation for Disabled people is a critical and non-negotiable component, which must hold equal with other vital elements of unlearning ableism. All people, whether they identify as Disabled or not, should have equity of access to opportunities and participation.

The equity of opportunity rhetoric is at the heart of the ambition to eradicate ableism. It stipulates that in an inclusive society, all individuals, Disabled or non-Disabled, are entitled to participate, contribute, and engage in the same manner through the creation of opportunity that bears no barriers. Equity of opportunity is a premise of positive action and active intervention, requiring the removal of material which may pose barriers to participation, contribution, and engagement for Disabled people.

Equity of opportunity secures fair competition, to ensure that individuals are able to compete and participate at the same level without the existence of unfair advantage, unfair treatment, accessibility barriers, or discrimination. Miller (1996) summarises the equity of opportunity rhetoric as 'equalising where people end up rather than where or how they begin'. Regardless of Disability (beginning), an individual is entitled to the same opportunities (ending), through the removal of equity of opportunity barriers such as financial implications, perceptions, and accessibility barriers. Encompassed within the equity of opportunity rhetoric is equality of process, perception, and autonomy. A Disabled person must be perceived as equal in value, worth, talent, and ability as a non-Disabled person. A Disabled person must be treated in the same non-discriminatory manner and receive fair treatment, process, and management as a non-Disabled person.

Now don't we all like the sound of this? The removal of Disability barriers to unlearn ableism is achieved through active intervention, promotion, and action, both individually and organisationally. We have to not only look within ourselves but also look within our structures and systems. The ongoing exclusion and neglecting of Disabled people by preventable accessibility barriers is ethically, economically, and socially damaging. But it can be broken. Through allyship, we can take action to break down ableism. To take action is to create equity of opportunity.

Allyship, as you can clearly tell, is a necessary building block in tackling ableism head on, creating unification and solidarity, leading to meaningful change and progress towards a more just and equitable world. We cannot do this on our own – we have for too long, and we have still so far to go to end the discrimination of Disabled people, so we need everyone to play their part.

> 66 As a neurodivergent person with over a decade of experience as a teacher and personal assistant to Disabled adults, and someone who now works alongside an incredible team of Disabled people every day, I believe that allyship is not passive – it's about action. It's about showing up, listening, and most importantly, creating tangible change. Too often, I see organisations talk about inclusion without taking the necessary steps to make it a reality. If we are serious about breaking down barriers, we must hold ourselves accountable and embed accessibility and inclusion into everything we do. At Happy Smiles Training, we don't just train people on Disability inclusion – we actively create employment and volunteering opportunities for Disabled people, ensuring

that the change we talk about starts from within. Over 92% of our workforce, from our advisory board to volunteers, have lived experience of Disability, and every session we deliver is designed and led by Disabled people. This isn't tokenism; I believe this is what meaningful action looks like.

Allyship is also about challenging the systems that hold Disabled people back. That means questioning outdated policies, fighting for fair wages for Disabled employees, and recognising that accessibility is a fundamental right, not a favour. It means celebrating Disabled people for their strengths, not their struggles. So, my challenge to anyone reading this chapter is: what action will you take today to create change? Because the difference between performative allyship and real impact is action. Let's be the change, together. 〞

– Alex Winstanely, Managing Director of Happy Smiles Training CIC

Carers and the role of allyship

Addressing ableism is a collective responsibility. It is not solely the duty of Disabled individuals to advocate for their rights; everyone, including carers, family members, friends, and the community, is playing a role in combating ableism and promoting accessibility (Kane, 2024).

Carers are often our first advocates: they fight on our behalf, they amplify our voices, and they can act as a bridge across the gap between Disabled people and broader societal systems. For many young Disabled people, parents and caregivers often provide an element of care for their Disabled child, being that rock, that source of support, that first line of defence.

66 As a child, Jamie's challenges were evident. I would match his socks because he couldn't see the difference between navy and black, lay out his clothes, help him with buttons and laces, and cut up his meals due to his struggles with hand-eye coordination. If I was meeting him outside school, I would describe my clothing to help him identify me. People assumed that wearing glasses would fix his vision or that because he wasn't visibly Disabled, he wasn't Disabled enough. A school psychologist even told me Jamie wouldn't suit specialist education because he didn't look like the other children.

There was no handbook, no support, no networks; I just had to get on with it. I was at the school nearly every week, fighting for the support he needed. Meetings led to let-downs, and although I managed to secure him a classroom assistant, he still struggled. Once, he came home covered in blood after walking into a gate unsupervised. The school sent him home like that, and I marched him straight back. Doctors would speak to me as if I didn't understand, but their advice often contradicted the specialists.

How do you explain to a child that they'll face barriers, that society won't support them like home does? By teaching them to accept and articulate their needs. I didn't know this was ableism; I had to learn from experience. My advice to other parents? Don't be intimidated by professionals. Trust your instincts. You know your child best. Let them find their own way. 99

– Tanya Devlin, mummy and past carer of Jamie Shields

Including carers in discussions about ableism and allyship is crucial – who better to understand and support than those who have supported us through it?

" Navigating the maze of the NHS is daunting, especially when you're juggling the complex realities of mental health issues or physical challenges. As a caregiver who has experienced these challenges, I've witnessed first-hand the gaps between the promise of care and the reality of service delivery. Big shout out for action, honesty, transparency, empathy, and accountability with open, clear communication within our broken healthcare system. My mum is an ex-midwife/sister, now living with dementia; it's an emotional rollercoaster for her, me, and our family. My mother also lives with rheumatoid arthritis, causing her to face daily physical limitations that impact all aspects of her life.

Mental health is another critical area where the promise of comprehensive care sometimes falls short. I've been battling depression. Having lost contact with my brother due to a system that has let us all down, I know all too well how delays in treatment, long waiting lists, and a lack of personalised care can ignite already difficult situations. I have witnessed how a system under pressure can sometimes overlook the silent battles people fight daily. This surely also impacts the workforce.

Accountability means ensuring that the vulnerable are not lost in the system and that every patient receives timely, compassionate care. Despite assurances from the local authority and NHS, the support often feels reactive and hurried rather than proactive and considered. We must collectively push for a system where transparency isn't an afterthought, where the voices of the most vulnerable are heard, and where accountability drives real change. "

**– Carl Nandoo, Disability access ambassador
and care advocate**

But how do we all play our part?

We need to use:

- respectful curiosity
- positive intention
- self-reflection and individual responsibility
- proactive, not reactive, practical responses
- a global, intersectional perspective.

In addition to the role that allyship plays and the importance of the actions of non-Disabled people, we cannot forget or fail to acknowledge the incredible work of those in the Disability community who throughout history have dedicated their lives to creating a better and more just world, those in the Disability movement who have paved the way for our generations now and our generations to come, those who have lost their lives at the hand of discrimination, those who have been pushed aside for their 'radical' beliefs, those who have achieved great change, and those who continue to do so.

It is because of them that we are here today, able to have these conversations, able to tap into the existing building blocks of change they created, with a chance to change the world.

How can we do better?

To be an ally and an active warrior of ableism, we must have three components. First, conscious positive intention. To act with intent is to act with a goal and an objective. We cannot be passive admirers from afar in the journey to unlearn ableism; we have to join in and play our part. The goal of eradicating ableism will only be achieved once every single one of us is part of the match. And we do this with a positive goal in mind, one that drives our actions, thoughts, and beliefs, one that shapes and moulds our minds in how we treat and care for others. We make a conscious choice to take action. Not once, but consistently.

Second, anticipatory duty. We act always with the acknowledgement of Disabled people. When we plan an event, we don't wait for a Disabled person to say they are coming; we assume they are. When we build a website, we don't wonder if Disabled people will visit; we build it assuming they will. When we recruit a new team member, we don't wait for a Disabled person to be unable to access the recruitment process; we make it accessible and inclusive from the start. Whether as an individual or an organisation, we all have a duty to involve Disabled people automatically, and by doing so we are working proactively to tear down barriers.

And third, and perhaps most importantly, a saying we have stated throughout this journey of unlearning: being proactive not reactive. Don't wait for a Disabled person to be discriminated against because they couldn't access your business, or website, or sports club, or job advert, or friendship group. Proactively from the start, ensure the elimination of ableism barriers. Being proactive not reactive also takes on a second meaning: to be proactive is to create or control a situation rather than react to it. Create a world of equity and inclusion, go and seek the blocks to tear down, go and find the walls to smash away, for all of us.

You might notice something missing here: 'nothing about us without us'. We're coming to it – it deserves a whole section on its own, and in a moment you will find out why.

Circling back again into accountability, our friend also plays another vital role in tackling ableism – consequence and repercussions, or in this case, a lack of. Despite a framework of international laws and the unanimous precedent to prevent discrimination, arguably one of the greatest reasons why the hamster wheel keeps on turning is because consequence is practically non-existent. Just 20.9% of Disabled people always feel comfortable to challenge ableism, and only 58.5% of Disabled people would definitely feel comfortable communicating their experiences about ableism (Disabled by Society, 2024).

As we know by now, Disabled people face multiple barriers, such as inaccessibility, bias, language, behaviours, attitudes, discrimination, beliefs, prejudice, segregation, and oppression. This creates an environment where Disabled people feel less able or willing to communicate their experiences or challenge behaviour for fear of repercussions, or lack of positive outcome. We know that when we call out behaviour or try to take action ourselves, a lot of the time we and not the perpetrator end up suffering the consequences. Why? People don't understand the law and what they shouldn't be doing, people don't understand the gravity of their actions, and people believe that justifications are acceptable.

For too long, ableism has been permitted in our society, without repercussions. Disabled people unanimously believe that not enough is being done to address ableism, with major failures in education, employment, government, and wider society to build awareness and introduce policies that break down barriers for Disabled people and eradicate misinformation. Ableism is out in the open for all to witness. Ableist behaviour is not being called out, prevented, or intervened with enough by non-Disabled people. Unlike other forms of discrimination, there is no set precedent or repercussions for ableist action. A lack of education and awareness has created a perpetual cycle where Disabled people feel isolated, face accessibility and attitudinal barriers, and are actively discriminated against, creating a cycle of justified ableism and internalised ableism.

Proactiveness and positive action are evidently inherently absent. Society must take positive action to create safe, open, and honest places of discussion that allow for the barriers of ableism to be broken down. Ableism has to be treated with the severity it deserves; to do this is to unlearn ableism.

From the point of design, we have to be getting it right. We have said that phrase quite a lot throughout this book, haven't we, so what does it actually mean and why is it so important? It means applying methods of design, thinking, action, principles, and practices that eradicate or are not inherently ableist from the very beginning when we are addressing any issue at hand.

In the context of allyship, as we spoke about earlier, it means looking at how we design principles and practices that can be utilised to create more inclusive and equitable solutions, involving products, services, systems, and experiences that are accessible for everyone, regardless of their background or identity, and involving Disabled people throughout the process. Imagine what the world would look and be like if we always thought about Disabled people in the decisions we took? Well, one day we hope we won't have to imagine. By adopting 'from the point of design' thinking, we will be more innovative and creative and be better at enacting positive conscious action, challenging systemic biases, and promoting the removal of Disability barriers. This is a valuable tool in creating meaningful and sustainable change.

> 66 Growing up with cerebral palsy, I didn't initially see myself as Disabled. My childhood dreams mirrored those of any other child until, around age eight or nine, societal attitudes, particularly regressive views within the South Asian community, began to highlight my differences. I was stereotyped and bullied; my

confidence waned, and so I suffered academically, not due
to ability but because I internalised the limits others imposed.
Yet leaving school marked a turning point – I resolved to chart
my own path. Music became my refuge. As a Bhangra singer,
I expressed myself beyond societal labels, performing and
connecting with others in ways that rendered my Disability
invisible. Little did I know that by my sheer presence on stage,
I was changing attitudes.

But when my music career ended, I faced another harsh reality:
unemployment. Despite my skills, I was judged again by my
impairment. Encouraged to volunteer at a Disability charity,
I initially felt boxed into a stereotype. Yet, the experience was
transformative. I saw how systemic barriers, not impairments,
held Disabled people back. This realisation fuelled my
determination to challenge norms. As a CEO, I became a living
example of a Disabled leader shaping policy and amplifying
voices in spaces often devoid of lived experience. To anyone
facing similar struggles, my advice is this: refuse to be defined
by others' perceptions. Create your own path, and when
obstacles arise, forge new ones. Change only happens with us
in the driving seat. 99

– Dr Amo Raju OBE

Nothing about us without us

Talking of phrases we have used over and over again in this book,
now we are reaching the end of this part of our journey, there is one
thing left to say, and a rather pertinent one at that: nothing about
us without us. Originating from the Latin *nihil de nobis, sine nobis*, it
means that nothing should be decided by any representative without

the full and direct participation of the members of a community affected by that decision.

The democratic theory of *nihil de nobis, sine nobis*, which was used throughout early European politics, was adopted by Disability advocates in the 1990s and by 2004 was the United Nations annual theme for the International Day of Persons with Disabilities. It is also now associated with the Convention on the Rights of Persons with Disabilities, which we learned about earlier. The best people to tell you what Disabled people want and need are Disabled people themselves; a world designed to be accessible for Disabled people cannot happen if Disabled people are not involved in the decision-making process.

We wouldn't set up a women's rights committee governed entirely by men, would we? So why do we think it acceptable to have decisions made about Disabled people, for Disabled people, without Disabled people? It isn't acceptable. Through our actions in unlearning ableism, we have to improve our engagement, consultation, and involvement of Disabled people from end-to-end. To achieve full participation and the equity of opportunity for Disabled people, the foundations of 'nothing about us without us' are critical, and encompass nearly everything we have learned and discussed throughout this book. Use our talents, highlight our skills, hear our voices, consult us, engage us; we hold the key to so many solutions that, when partnered together through the powers of allyship, are our tools to breaking down barriers.

We like to call them the big three Cs: through *consistency*, *collaboration*, and *creativity*, ableism can be a thing of the past. Work with us not against us, we cannot be ignored any longer – everything is about us so let nothing be without us.

So there we are...we have reached the end, and as we draw this chapter to a close, what have we learned? That change does not come from being passive; change comes from positive, conscious action, whether as allies or as a Disabled person ourselves. Change comes from you taking what you have learned, bringing it into the world, and sharing that knowledge! Mahatma Gandhi famously said, 'Be the change that you wish to see in the world.' And now, you know how.

There is a very good reason we left this particular chapter until last – because as you have probably guessed, it is the cherry on top of the sundae, a synopsis of everything we have been discussing, giving you the actionable tools as you close these final pages to think differently moving forward.

Ableism is inherently aggressive in its nature; it will not stop of its own accord, it will continue and grow if the antidotes are not administered. We must challenge ableism at both the individual and systemic levels, working towards creating a more inclusive and equitable world for all.

Unlearning ableism starts with you.

As Francis of Assisi said, 'Start by doing what's necessary; then do what's possible; and suddenly you are doing the impossible.' We are necessary, and we are here to do the impossible.

References

Accenture, Disability:IN, and the American Association of People with Disabilities. (2018). *Getting to Equal: The Disability Inclusion Advantage.* www.accenture.com/content/dam/accenture/final/a-com-migration/pdf/pdf-89/accenture-disability-inclusion-research-report.pdf

Access2Funding. (2023). *Access2Funding 2023 Report. Transforming Opportunities & Outcomes for Disabled Entrepreneurs.* www.linkedin.com/posts/access2fundingcic_access2funding-2023-report-activity-7089193215102201856-3e4V

American Psychiatric Association. (2024). *Stigma, Prejudice and Discrimination Against People with Mental Illness.* www.psychiatry.org/patients-families/stigma-and-discrimination

American Psychological Association. (2020). *Stress in America: The Impact of COVID-19 on Mental Health.* www.apa.org/news/press/releases/stress/2020/sia-mental-health-crisis.pdf

Americans with Disabilities Act (ADA) 1990, United States. (1990). US Department of Justice.

Ames, S.G, Delaney, R.K, Houtrow, A.J., *et al.* (2023). Perceived Disability-based discrimination in healthcare for children with medical complexity and Disability. *Pediatrics*, 152(1), e2022060975. https://doi.org/10.1542/peds.2022-060975

Amoakuh, A. (2024). *Europe still sterilises disabled women despite the practice being a human rights violation.* Screenshot. https://screenshot-media.com/politics/human-rights/disabled-women-sterilised-europe

Anderson, S. (2020). *A Cultural History of Disability in The Renaissance. Social*

History Society. https://socialhistory.org.uk/shs_exchange/a-cultural-history-of-disability-in-the-renaissance

Anti-Bullying Alliance. (2019). *Tackling Disablist Language Based Bullying in School: A Teacher's Guide*. https://anti-bullyingalliance.org.uk/sites/default/files/uploads/attachments/tackling-disablist-language-based-bullying-in-school-final.pdf

Atkins Jacob. (2022). *Reference Wheelchair Research: Full Report*. Department for Transport. https://assets.publishing.service.gov.uk/media/6230946ce90e070ed04a1d6f/reference-wheelchair-report.pdf

Australian Bureau of Statistics. (2020). *Disability and the Labour Force*. www.abs.gov.au/articles/disability-and-labour-force

Barnes, C. & Mercer, G. (2004). *Disability Policy and Practice: Applying the Social Model*. Leeds: The Disability Press.

Bascom, J. (2019). *Position Statement on Applied Behavior Analysis (ABA)*. Autistic Self Advocacy Network.

BBC Newsround. (2023). What is Disability Pride Month? www.bbc.co.uk/newsround/6625633.

BMC Health Services Research. (2021). Racial and ethnic disparities in healthcare access and quality for people with disabilities. *BMC Health Services Research*, 21(1), 1–9.

Braich, A. (2021). *Why Family Caregivers are Likely to Develop PTSD*. Camino Recovery. www.caminorecovery.com/blog/why-family-caregivers-are-likely-to-develop-ptsd

Broberg, G. & Tydén, M. (2005). *Eugenics in Sweden: Efficient Care*. Michigan State University Press.

Business Disability Forum. (2023). *The Great Big Workplace Adjustments Survey 2023*. https://businessdisabilityforum.org.uk/gbwas-what-did-people-tell-us

Business Disability Forum. (2024). *Disabled people often not seen in media and advertising content, new research finds*. https://businessdisabilityforum.org.uk/disabled-people-not-seen-in-images-new-research-finds

Business Disability Forum. (2025). *Disability Awareness Days*. https://businessdisabilityforum.org.uk/about-us/media-centre/disability-awareness-dates

Cambridge Dictionary. (n.d.b). *Entrepreneur*. https://dictionary.cambridge.org/dictionary/english/entrepreneur

Cambridge Dictionary. (n.d.c). *Legislation*. https://dictionary.cambridge.org/dictionary/learner-english/legislation

Cambridge Dictionary. (n.d.). *Policy*. https://dictionary.cambridge.org/dictionary/english/policy

Cambridge Dictionary. (n.d.). *Privilege*. https://dictionary.cambridge.org/dictionary/english/privilege

Care Quality Commission. (2020). *Protect, Respect, Connect – Decisions about Living and Dying Well During COVID-19*. www.cqc.org.uk/publications/themed-work/protect-respect-connect-decisions-about-living-dying-well-during-covid-19

Carers UK. (2023). *Carers' Employment Rights Today, Tomorrow and in the Future*. www.carersuk.org/media/hiekwx0p/carers-uk-crd-employment-report-2023_final.pdf

CCBlogC. (2019). *The Numbers Are In: 2019 CCBC Diversity Statistics*. https://ccblogc.blogspot.com/2020/06/the-numbers-are-in-2019-ccbc-diversity.html

Centers for Disease Control and Prevention. (2023). *Disability Impacts all of Us Infographic*. www.cdc.gov/disability-and-health/articles-documents/disability-impacts-all-of-us-infographic.html

Centers for Disease Control and Prevention. (2024). *The Mental Health of People with Disabilities*. www.cdc.gov/disability-and-health/articles-documents/mental-health-of-people-with-disabilities.html

Centre for Social Justice. (2021). *Now is the Time. A report by the CSJ Disability Commission*. www.centreforsocialjustice.org.uk/wp-content/uploads/2021/03/CSJJ8819-Disability-Report-190408.pdf

Chowdhury, R., Furst, L., & Sharma, V. (2020). Health disparities in the U.S. disabled population: Understanding the challenges of access and care. *Journal of Health Disparities Research and Practice*, 13(3), 45–59. https://pmc.ncbi.nlm.nih.gov/articles/PMC10357509

Cimpean, D. & Drake, R.E. (2011). Treating co-morbid medical conditions and anxiety/depression. *Epidemiology and Psychiatric Sciences*, 20(2), 141–150.

Claricoats, L. (2024). *Barriers into Higher Education for Disabled Students: A Literature Review*. Sheffield Hallam University. https://shura.shu.ac.uk/33456/1/Claricoats_2024_barriers_into_higher_education.pdf

Community Care. (2021). *Social care cuts and increased charges causing huge distress for disabled people*. www.communitycare.co.uk/2021/04/13/social-care-cuts-increased-charges-causing-huge-distress-disabled-people

Concern Worldwide. (2023, June 19). *The Vicious Cycle of Poverty Explained*. www.concern.org.uk/news/vicious-cycle-poverty-explained

Corrigan, P.W. & Watson, A.C. (2002). The paradox of self-stigma and mental illness. *Clinical Psychology: Science and Practice*, 9(1), 35–53. https://doi.org/10.1093/clipsy.9.1.35

Council of Europe. (1950). *European Convention on Human Rights*. https://www.echr.coe.int/documents/d/echr/convention_ENG

Cree, R.A., Okoro, C.A., Zack, M.M., & Carbone, E. (2020). Frequent mental distress among adults, by disability status, disability type, and selected characteristics – United States, 2018. *Morbidity & Mortality Weekly Report*, 69, 1238–1243. www.cdc.gov/mmwr/volumes/69/wr/mm6936a2.htm?s_cid=mm6936a2_w

Crenshaw, K.W. (1989). Demarginalizing the intersection of race and sex: A Black feminist critique of antidiscrimination doctrine, feminist theory, and antiracist politics. *University of Chicago Legal Forum*, 1989(1), 139–167. https://chicagounbound.uchicago.edu/uclf/vol1989/iss1/8

Cunnington, R. (2019). *Neuroplasticity: How the Brain Changes with Learning*. International Bureau of Education, UNESCO. https://solportal.ibe-unesco.org/articles/neuroplasticity-how-the-brain-changes-with-learning

de Castro, C. (2024). *Disability in the Fashion Industry: Beyond Tokenism to True Inclusion*. Purple Goat Agency. www.purplegoatagency.com/insights/disability-in-the-fashion-industry

Deloitte. (2024). *Disability Inclusion @ Work 2024: A Global Outlook*. www.deloitte.com/global/en/issues/work/content/disability-inclusion-at-work.html

Demony, C. (2024). *Campaigners Seek EU-wide Ban on Forced Sterilisation of People with Disabilities*. Reuters. www.reuters.com/world/europe/campaigners-seek-eu-wide-ban-forced-sterilisation-people-with-disabilities-2024-04-12

Department for Education. (2020a). *School Snapshot Survey: Summer 2019*. Gov.uk www.gov.uk/government/publications/school-snapshot-survey-summer-2019

Department for Education. (2020b). *Special Educational Needs in England: Academic Year 2019/20*. Gov.uk. https://explore-education-statistics.service.gov.uk/find-statistics/special-educational-needs-in-england/2019-20

Department for Work and Pensions. (2022). *Disability Confident Scheme: Findings from a survey of participating employers*. Gov.uk. https://assets.publishing.service.gov.uk/media/64db611cc8dee4000d7f1c95/disability-confident-members-survey-report-2022.pdf

Department for Work and Pensions. (2023). *Family Resources Survey: Financial Year 2021 to 2022*. Gov.uk. www.gov.uk/government/statistics/family-resources-survey-financial-year-2021-to-2022

Disability Horizons. (2022). *Less than 2% of characters in the top UK TV shows are disabled*. https://disabilityhorizons.com/2022/10/less-than-2-of-characters-in-the-top-uk-tv-show-are-disabled

Disability Nottinghamshire. (n.d.). *Social Model vs Medical Model of Disability*. www.disabilitynottinghamshire.org.uk/index.php/about/social-model-vs-medical-model-of-disability

Disability Office. (2021). *Using a Range of Communication Channels to Reach Disabled People*. www.gov.uk/government/publications/inclusive-communication/using-a-range-of-communication-channels-to-reach-disabled-people

Disability Rights Education and Defense Fund. (2020). *The Illegality of Medical Rationing on the Basis of Disability*. https://dredf.org/wp-content/uploads/2020/03/DREDF-Policy-Statement-on-COVID-19-and-Medical-Rationing-3-25-2020.pdf

Disability Rights Education and Defense Fund. (2025). *History of the Independent Living Movement*.

Disability Rights UK. (2022a). *Disability Rights UK Hate Crime Charter: Tackling Everyday Hate Against Disabled People*. www.disabilityrightsuk.org/system/files/paragraphs/cw_file/2023-04/Accessible%20word%20doc%20-%20Disability%20Hate%20Crime%20Charter%20-%20Disability%20Rights%20UK%202022.docx

Disability Rights UK. (2022b). *Disabled People Make Up Nearly Half of the Most Deprived Working-Age Adults in the Country*. www.disabilityrightsuk.org/news/2022/july/disabled-people-make-nearly-half-most-deprived-working-age-adults-country

Disability Unit UK. (2021). *UK Disability Survey Research Report, June 2021*. Gov.uk. www.gov.uk/government/publications/uk-disability-survey-research-report-june-2021/uk-disability-survey-research-report-june-2021

Disability:IN. (2023). *2023 Disability Index Report*. https://disabilityin.org/2023-dei-report

Disabled by Society. (2024, July). *The Big Ableism Survey Policy Paper*. https://disabledbysociety.com/disabled-by-society-resources/

Eisenmenger, E. (2020). *Five Things You Didn't Know About Invisible Disabilities*. Access Living. www.accessliving.org/newsroom/blog/five-things-you-didnt-know-about-invisible-disabilities

EU Employment Equality Directive (2000/78/EC), European Union. (2000). http://data.europa.eu/eli/dir/2000/78/oj

European Foundation for the Improvement of Living and Working Conditions. (2021). *European Quality of Life Surveys.* www.eurofound.europa.eu/en/surveys/european-quality-life-surveys-eqls

European Parliament (2020). *Employment and disability in the European Union.* (EPRS PE 651.932). https://www.europarl.europa.eu/RegData/etudes/BRIE/2020/651932/EPRS_BRI(2020)651932_EN.pdf

European Union Agency for Fundamental Rights. (2020). *Employment and Disability in the European Union.* www.europarl.europa.eu/RegData/etudes/BRIE/2020/651932/EPRS_BRI(2020)651932_EN.pdf

Eurostat. (2024). *Statistics Explained.* https://ec.europa.eu/eurostat/statistics-explained/index.php?title=Population_with_disability&utm

Evans, J. (2003). *The Independent Living Movement in the UK.* Independent Living Institute. www.independentliving.org/docs6/evans2003.html

Evenbreak. (2020). *The Real Barriers to Employment Faced by Disabled People.* https://blog.evenbreak.co.uk/2020/03/03/the-real-barriers-to-employment-faced-by-disabled-people/

Family Caregiver Alliance. (n.d.). *Caregiver Statistics: Health, Technology, and Caregiving Resources.* www.caregiver.org/resource/caregiver-statistics-health-technology-and-caregiving-resources

Fenney, D. (2023). *Tackling Ableism in Health Care – The Role of Primary Care.* The King's Fund. www.kingsfund.org.uk/insight-and-analysis/blogs/tackling-ableism-health-care

Fox, L. (2020). *Supplemental Poverty Measure: 2019.* US Census Bureau. www.census.gov/library/publications/2020/demo/p60-272.html

Friedlander, H. (1995). *The Origins of Nazi Genocide: From Euthanasia to the Final Solution.* University of North Carolina Press.

Friedman, C. (2024). *Many Disability Professionals Don't Understand Ableism.* The Council on Quality and Leadership. www.c-q-l.org/resources/articles/many-disability-professionals-dont-understand-ableism

Gevorkian, D. (2024). *The Cost of Inaccessibility: Businesses Lose More than $6.9 Billion Annually.* Retail TouchPoints. www.retailtouchpoints.com/features/executive-viewpoints/the-cost-of-inaccessibility-businesses-lose-more-than-6-9-billion-annually

Golightley, M. & Holloway, M. (2016). Editorial. *The British Journal of Social Work*, 46(1), 1–7. https://academic.oup.com/bjsw/article-abstract/46/1/1/2495107?redirectedFrom=fulltext

Gonzalez, D., Kenney, G.M., Karpman, M, & Morriss, S. (2023). *Four in Ten Adults with Disabilities Experienced Unfair Treatment in Health Care Settings, at Work, or When Applying for Public Benefits in 2022.* Urban Institute. www. urban.org/research/publication/four-ten-adults-disabilities-experienced-unfair-treatment-health-care-settings

Governor's Council on Developmental Disabilities. (2025). *Parallels in Time: A History of Developmental Disabilities.* https://mn.gov/mnddc/parallels

Harris, J. (2025, 19 January). Shut away and ignored: Thousands of disabled adults are at the mercy of a broken system. *The Guardian.* www. theguardian.com/commentisfree/2025/jan/19/millions-shut-out-society-social-care-crisis-disabled-adults

Hatton, J. (2020). *The Real Barriers to Employment Faced by Disabled People.* Evenbreak. https://blog.evenbreak.co.uk/2020/03/03/the-real-barriers-to-employment-faced-by-disabled-people

Herr, S. (2016). Representation of clients with disabilities: Issues of ethics and control. *N.Y.U Review of Law & Social Change*, 17(4). https://socialchangenyu.com/review/representation-of-clients-with-disabilities-issues-of-ethics-and-control

Historic England. (2024). *Building Regulations, Approved Documents and Historic Buildings.* https://historicengland.org.uk/advice/technical-advice/building-regulations/?utm_

Historic England. (2025). *History of Disability: From 1050 to the Present Day.* https://historicengland.org.uk/research/inclusive-heritage/disability-history

HRC Foundation. (2022). *Understanding Disability in the LGBTQ+ Community.* www.hrc.org/resources/understanding-disabled-lgbtq-people

Iezzoni, L.I., Rao, S.R., Ressalam, J., Bolcic-Jankovic, D., *et al.* (2021). Physicians' perceptions of people with disability and their health care. *Health Affairs*, 40(2), 297–306. https://doi.org/10.1377/hlthaff.2020.01452

Inclusion Canada. (n.d.). *11 Interesting Facts about the CRPD.* https://inclusioncanada.ca/2022/03/04/11-interesting-facts-about-the-crpd

Inclusion London. (2025). *Barriers at Home: Housing Crisis for Deaf and Disabled Londoners.* www.inclusionlondon.org.uk/services-and-support/our-projects/disability-and-housing-in-london/barriers-at-home

Inevitable Foundation. (2024). *Audiences Are Waiting for Hollywood to Greenlight Disability: A Survey on Disability and Mental Health Representation in Film and TV.* www.inevitable.foundation/press/deadline-greenlight

International Alliance of Carer Organizations. (2021). *Global Carer Stats.* International Carers.org. https://internationalcarers.org/carer-facts/global-carer-stats

International Labour Organisation. (2018). *World Employment and Social Outlook – Disability and Work*. www.ilo.org/publications/world-employment-and-social-outlook-trends-2018

International Paralympic Committee. (2025). *Paralympics History*. www.paralympic.org/ipc/history

James, S.E., Herman, J.L., Rankin, S., & Keisling, M. (2013). *The Report of the 2011 National Transgender Discrimination Survey*. National Center for Transgender Equality and the National Gay and Lesbian Task Force.

Jammaers, E. & Fleischmann, A. (2024). Unveiling affective disablism at work: A structural approach to microaggressions. *Disability & Society*, 40(6), 1622–1645. https://doi.org/10.1080/09687599.2024.2368561

Jarret, S. (2023). *A History of Disability in England from the Medieval Period to the Present Day*. Liverpool University Press, Historic England.

Jenkins, R. (2024). Millions with a disability feel left out by retailers who ignore accessibility needs. *The Sun*. www.thesun.co.uk/money/31681734/millions-disability-retailers-left-out-accessibility

Jerez, M. (2024). *Accessibility in social media: Do's and don'ts* [Webinar]. https://ec.europa.eu/regional_policy/sources/policy/communication/webinar/Social_media_accessibility_nov24.pdf

Job Accommodation Network. (2024). *Costs and Benefits of Accommodation*. https://askjan.org/topics/costs.cfm

John Smith Centre. (2023). *The Political Representation of Disabled People and People with Long-Term Health Conditions Across the United Kingdom*. www.johnsmithcentre.com/research-blog/the-political-representation-of-disabled-people

Kadja, K., Marx, A., Richards, J.D., *et al.* (2017). Archaeology, heritage, and social value: Public perspectives on European archaeology. *European Journal of Archaeology*, 2(1), 96–117. https://doi.org/10.1017/eaa.2017.19

Kane, S. (2024). *Understanding Ableism: A Call to Action for Social Justice*. Inside Networks. www.insidenetworks.org/2024/09/26/understanding-ableism-a-call-to-action-for-social-justice

Kearl, H. (2010). *Stop Street Harassment: Making Public Places Safe and Welcoming for Women*. Praeger Publishers.

Keierleber, M. (2019). *Report: Most Students With Learning Disabilities Learn in General Ed Classrooms, but Few Teachers Feel Confident in Their Ability to Teach Them*. The 74. https://www.the74million.org/report-most-students-with-learning-disabilities-learn-in-general-ed-classrooms-but-few-teachers-feel-confident-in-their-ability-to-teach-them

Kelly, R. & Mutebi, N. (2023). *Invisible Disabilities in Education and Employment*. Post Parliament. https://post.parliament.uk/research-briefings/post-pn-0689

Kuehn, B.M. (2010). Gender differences in ADHD diagnosis and treatment. *JAMA*, 304(6), 636–638.

Lagu, T., Griffin, C., Donelan, K., & Iezzoni, L.I. (2022). I am not the doctor for you: Physicians' attitudes about caring for people with disabilities. *Health Affairs*, 41(10), 1387–1396. https://doi.org/10.1377/hlthaff.2022.00475

Le, D., Ozbeki, H., Salazar, S., Berl, M., Turner, M.M., & Acosta Price, O. (2022). Improving African American women's engagement in clinical research: A systematic review of barriers to participation in clinical trials. *Journal of the National Medical Association*, 114(3), 324–339.

Leonard Cheshire. (2022). *Rising costs are a catastrophe for disabled people*. www.leonardcheshire.org/about-us/our-news/press-releases/rising-costs-are-catastrophe-disabled-people

Maker, Y. (2022). 'Disability Rights and Carers' Advocacy.' In *Care and Support Rights After Neoliberalism*. Cambridge University Press.

Maloney, W. (2017). *World War I: Injured Veterans and the Disability Rights Movement*. Library of Congress Blogs. https://blogs.loc.gov/loc/2017/12/world-war-i-injured-veterans-and-the-disability-rights-movement

Martini, M.I., Kuja-Halkola, R., Butwicka, A., Du Rietz, E. *et al.* (2025). Sex differences in psychiatric diagnoses preceding autism diagnosis and their stability post autism diagnosis. *Journal of Child Psychology and Psychiatry*. https://doi.org/10.1111/jcpp.14130

Maroto, M.L. & Pettinicchio, D. (2022). *Disability and Economic Precarity. The Gender Policy Report*. University of Minnesota. https://genderpolicyreport.umn.edu/disability-and-economic-precarity

Mazzeo, E. (2025). *As the LA wildfires have shown, people with disabilities often have to fend for themselves*. CNN. https://edition.cnn.com/2025/01/18/health/disability-la-fire-evacuations-wellness/index.html

McTernan, E. (2018). Microaggressions, equality, and social practices. *Journal of Political Philosophy*, 26(3), 261–281. https://doi.org/10.1111/jopp.12150

Meldon, P. (2015). *Disability History: The Disability Rights Movement*. National Park Service. www.nps.gov/articles/disabilityhistoryrightsmovement.htm

Mencap. (n.d.). *Children – research and statistics*. www.mencap.org.uk/learning-disability-explained/research-and-statistics/children-research-and-statistics

Mental Health Foundation. (2021). *Stigma and discrimination*. https://www.mentalhealth.org.uk/explore-mental-health/a-z-topics/stigma-and-discrimination

Miller, D. (1996). Two cheers for meritocracy. *The Journal of Political Philosophy*, 4(4), 277–301. https://doi.org/10.1111/j.1467-9760.1996.tb00053.x

Miserandino, C. (2003). *The Spoon Theory*. Butyoudontlooksick.com. www.butyoudontlooksick.com/articles/written-by-christine/the-spoon-theory

Mitchell, D. (2003). A chapter in the history of nurse education: Learning disability nursing and The Jay Report. *Nurse Education Today*, 23(5), 350–356. https://doi.org/10.1016/S0260-6917(03)00025-X

Moyo, T. (2020). Healthcare in South Africa: A study of access and quality in private vs. public systems. *South African Medical Review*, 12(3), 204–215.

Murphy, K. (2024). *Disability – A Brief Historical Overview*. San Diego State University. https://accessibility.sdsu.edu/news/disability-timeline

National Autistic Society. (n.d.). *What is Autism?* www.autism.org.uk/advice-and-guidance/what-is-autism

National Autistic Society. (2024). *ITV Investigation Highlights Broken SEND System*. www.autism.org.uk/what-we-do/news/itv-investigation-highlights-broken-send-system

National Autistic Society. (2025). *Empowering Autistic Travel*. www.motabilityfoundation.org.uk/media/nhbbgz0e/eat-research-report-26-mar-25-1708.pdf

National Bureau of Statistics of China. (2024). Statistical Communiqué of the People's Republic of China on the 2023 National Economic and Social Development. https://en.planning.org.cn/planning/view?id=1352

National Disability Institute. (2019a). *Race, Ethnicity and Disability: The Financial Impact of Systemic Inequality and Intersectionality*. www.nationaldisabilityinstitute.org/reports/research-brief-race-ethnicity-and-disability

National Disability Institute. (2019b). *Financial Inequality: Disability, Race and Poverty in America*. www.nationaldisabilityinstitute.org/wp-content/uploads/2019/02/disability-race-poverty-in-america.pdf

National Disability Institute. (2020). *The Extra Costs of Living with a Disability in the United States*. www.nationaldisabilityinstitute.org/reports/extra-costs-living-with-disability

National Education Union. (2024). *EPI Annual Report*. https://neu.org.uk/latest/press-releases/epi-annual-report-2024?

National Health Interview Survey. (2020). *Disability and Health: Access to Care and Costs*. Centers for Disease Control and Prevention. www.cdc.gov/nchs/nhis/index.html

National Institutes of Health. (2023). *NIH Designates People with Disabilities as a Population with Health Disparities*. www.nih.gov/news-events/news-releases/nih-designates-people-disabilities-population-health-disparities

Ndugga, N., Hill, L., & Artiga, S. (2024). *Key Data on Health and Health Care by Race and Ethnicity*. Kaiser Family Foundation. www.kff.org/key-data-on-health-and-health-care-by-race-and-ethnicity/?utm_

Ndugga, N., Hill, L., Artiga, S., & Damico, A. (2025). *Health Coverage by Race and Ethnicity, 2010–2023*. Kaiser Family Foundation. www.kff.org/racial-equity-and-health-policy/issue-brief/health-coverage-by-race-and-ethnicity/?utm_

NHS Employers. (2023). *Making Workplace Adjustments to Support Disabled Staff*. www.nhsemployers.org/publications/making-workplace-adjustments-support-disabled-staff

NHS England. (n.d.). *NHS History*. www.england.nhs.uk/nhsbirthday/about-the-nhs-birthday/nhs-history

Nielsen. (2022). *Seen on Screen: The Importance of Disability Representation*. www.nielsen.com/insights/2022/the-importance-of-disability-representation

Office for Health Improvement & Disparities. (2022). *Abortion Statistics, England and Wales: 2022*. Gov.uk. www.gov.uk/government/statistics/abortion-statistics-for-england-and-wales-2022/abortion-statistics-england-and-wales-2022

Office for National Statistics. (2019). *Disability and Education, UK: 2019*. www.ons.gov.uk/peoplepopulationandcommunity/healthandsocialcare/disability/bulletins/disabilityandeducationuk/2019

Office for National Statistics. (2021). *Outcomes for Disabled People in the UK: 2020*. www.ons.gov.uk/peoplepopulationandcommunity/healthandsocialcare/disability/articles/outcomesfordisabledpeopleintheuk/2020

Office for National Statistics. (2022a). *Outcomes for Disabled People in the UK: 2021*. www.ons.gov.uk/peoplepopulationandcommunity/healthandsocialcare/disability/articles/outcomesfordisabledpeopleintheuk/2021

Office for National Statistics. (2022b). *Disability and Employment: A Statistical Overview*. www.ons.gov.uk/peoplepopulationandcommunity/healthandsocialcare/disability/datasets/disabilityandemployment

Office of Rail and Road. (2025). *Rail Passenger Assists 2024–25 Periods 5 to 7 (21 July 2024 to 12 October 2024)*. https://dataportal.orr.gov.uk/media/kcwfwsfe/assists-factsheet-2024-25-rail-periods-5-7.pdf

Okoro, C.A., Hollis, N.D., Cyrus, A.C., & Griffin-Blake, S. (2018). Prevalence of disabilities and health care access by disability status and type among adults – United States, 2016. *Morbidity & Mortality Weekly Report*, 67(32), 882–887. https://doi.org/10.15585/mmwr.mm6732a3

Oliver, M. (1983). *Social Work with Disabled People*. Macmillan.

Oswald, L. & Penketh, K. (2021). Challenging the motherhood myth: Perceptions of disabled women and parenting. *Frontiers in Psychology*, 12, Article 734041.

Oxford English Dictionary. (n.d.a). *Ableism*. www.oed.com/dictionary/ableism_n

Oxford English Dictionary. (n.d.). *Allyship*. www.oed.com/dictionary/allyship_n

Oxford English Dictionary. (n.d.c). *Discrimination*. www.oed.com/dictionary/discrimination_n

Oxford Review. (n.d.). *Ableism – Definition and Explanation*. https://oxford-review.com/the-oxford-review-dei-diversity-equity-and-inclusion-dictionary/ableism-definition-and-explanation

Patel, R. (2022). The state of public healthcare in India: Challenges and opportunities. *Indian Journal of Health Economics*, 39(4), 102–115.

Pring, J. (2019). *The Shocking Truth about Disability Benefits: Successful Appeals Double in a Decade*. Disability News Service. www.disabilitynewsservice.com/the-shocking-truth-about-disability-benefits-successful-appeals-double-in-a-decade

Psych Central. (2022). *ADHD in Women vs. Men: Does Gender Play a Role in Symptoms?* https://psychcentral.com/adhd/adhd-and-gender#diagnosis

Purple. (n.d.). *The Purple Pound Infographic*. https://wearepurple.org.uk/download/the-purple-pound-infographic

Raleigh, V. & Holmes, J. (2023). *The Health of People from Ethnic Minority Groups in England*. The King's Fund. www.kingsfund.org.uk/insight-and-analysis/long-reads/health-people-ethnic-minority-groups-england

Ratliff, K.A. & Tucker Smith, C. (2024). The Implicit Association Test. *Daedalus*, 153 (1), 51–64. https://doi.org/10.1162/daed_a_02048

Real Estate Investor Pulse. (2023, 5 July). *Less than 5% of American Homes Are Accessible for the Disabled and Elderly*. www.housingwire.com/articles/less-than-5-of-american-homes-are-accessible-for-the-disabled-elderly

ReliefWeb. (2024). *Protecting persons with disabilities, the forgotten victims of humanitarian crises.* https://reliefweb.int/report/world/protecting-persons-disabilities-forgotten-victims-humanitarian-crises

Reynolds, J.M. (2018). Three things clinicians should know about disability. *AMA Journal of Ethics*, December. doi: 10.1001/amajethics.2018.1181

Royal College of Nursing. (2025). *A History of Care or Control?* www.rcn.org.uk/library-exhibitions/Learning-disability-2020

Royal National Institute of Blind People. (2022). *Voice of the Customer Report: Travel and Transport.* www.rnib.org.uk/documents/2206/Voice_of_the_Customer_Report_-_Travel_and_Transport_2022.docx

Scope. (n.d.a). *Disability Facts and Figures.* www.scope.org.uk/media/disability-facts-figures

Scope (n.d.b). *Disability in the Workplace: How to Retain Disabled Staff in Employment.* www.scope.org.uk/campaigns/research-policy/employee-retention

Scope. (n.d.c). *Understanding the Challenges of Disabled Jobseekers.* https://business.scope.org.uk/understanding-the-challenges-of-disabled-jobseekers

Scope. (2014). *Brits feel uncomfortable with disabled people.* https://www.scope.org.uk/media/press-releases/brits-feel-uncomfortable-with-disabled-people

Scope. (2022). *Attitudes Research.* www.scope.org.uk/campaigns/research-policy/attitudes-towards-disabled-people

Scope. (2024). *Disability Price Tag 2024.* www.scope.org.uk/campaigns/disability-price-tag

Sense. (n.d.). *The Social Model of Disability.* www.sense.org.uk/about-us/the-social-model-of-disability

Shapiro, J.P. (1993). *No Pity: People with Disabilities Forging a New Civil Rights Movement.* Random House.

Sharma, R. (2021). *News by Numbers: Only 36% of India's 26 Million Persons with Disabilities are Employed.* Forbes India. www.forbesindia.com/article/news-by-numbers/news-by-numbers-only-36-of-indias-26-million-persons-with-disabilities-are-employed/68441/1

Shewan Stevens, H. (2024). 'The more help I needed, the more I had to beg for it': Disabled women are still the forgotten victims of domestic abuse. *Glamour Magazine.* www.glamourmagazine.co.uk/article/disabled-women-domestic-abuse

Shuman, T. (2025). *Family Caregiver Annual Report and Statistics*. Seniorliving. org. www.seniorliving.org/research/family-caregiver-report-statistics

Skills for Care. (2022). *The State of the Adult Social Care Sector and Workforce in England*. www.skillsforcare.org.uk/Adult-Social-Care-Workforce-Data/ Workforce-intelligence/documents/State-of-the-adult-social-care-sector/ The-state-of-the-adult-social-care-sector-and-workforce-2022.pdf

Smith, J. (2023). Private healthcare and government-funded programs in the United States: A comprehensive overview. *Health Policy Journal*, 45(2), 113–126.

Smith, S.G., Zhang, X., Basile, K.C., *et al.* (2021). The National Intimate Partner and Sexual Violence Survey (NISVS): 2019 State Report. *Psychological Trauma: Theory, Research, Practice, and Policy*, 13(3), 251–260.

Smith, S.L., Choueiti, M., & Pieper, K. (2016). *Inequality in 800 popular films: Examining portrayals of gender, race/ethnicity, LGBT, and disability from 2007 to 2015*. USC Annenberg School for Communication and Journalism. https://annenberg.usc.edu/sites/default/files/2017/04/10/MDSCI_ Inequality_in_800_Films_FINAL.pdf

Statistics Canada. (2023). *Labour Force Survey, 2022*. www150.statcan.gc.ca/n1/ daily-quotidien/230830/dq230830a-eng.htm

Statistics Canada. (2024). *Canadian Survey on Disability: 2022/2023 Results*. www150.statcan.gc.ca/n1/pub/89-654-x/89-654-x2024001-eng.htm

Stern, A. (2005). *Eugenic Nation: Faults and Frontiers of Better Breeding in Modern America*. University of California Press.

Temple University Institute on Disabilities. (n.d.). *Disability Rights Timeline*. https://disabilities.temple.edu/resources/disability-rights-timeline

The Open University. (2025). *Timeline of Learning Disability History*. https:// university.open.ac.uk/health-and-social-care/research/shld/timeline- learning-disability-history

The Trevor Project. (2023). *The Trevor Project Mental Health of LGBTQ+ Young People with Disabilities Report*. www.thetrevorproject.org/research-briefs/ the-mental-health-of-lgbtq-young-people-with-disabilities

The Trevor Project. (2024). *2024 U.S. National Survey on the Mental Health of LGBTQ+ Young People*. www.thetrevorproject.org/survey-2024

The Valuable 500. (2021). *Making Employment Accessible for People with Disabilities. The Valuable 500 Global Trends Report: Issue 6*. www. thevaluable500.com/wp-content/uploads/2021/11/V500_Global-Trends- Report_Issue-6_Designed-V7_FINAL.pdf

Thompson, J.E., Panella, S., Soncin, S., *et al.* (2025). The use-life of ancestors: Neolithic cranial retention, caching and disposal at Masseria Candelaro, Apulia, Italy. *European Journal of Archaeology*, 28(1), 3–23. doi:10.1017/eaa.2024.43

Titone, J. (2024). Absence of Special Olympics from 2024 Paris Games illustrates ableism in sport: Brock expert. *The Brock News*. https://brocku.ca/brock-news/2024/08/absence-of-special-olympics-from-2024-paris-games-illustrates-ableism-in-sport-brock-expert

UK Government. (n.d.). *Access to Work*. www.gov.uk/access-to-work

UK Government. (1998). *Human Rights Act 1998*. www.legislation.gov.uk/ukpga/1998/42/contents

UK Government. (2010). *Equality Act 2010*. www.gov.uk/definition-of-disability-under-equality-act-2010

UK Government. (2015). *Access to and use of buildings: Approved Document M*. www.gov.uk/government/publications/access-to-and-use-of-buildings-approved-document-m

UK Government. (2023). *Disability Confident: Employer Guide. Department for Work and Pensions*. www.gov.uk/government/collections/disability-confident-campaign

UK Parliament. (1995). *The Code of Conduct for Members of Parliament*. https://publications.parliament.uk/pa/cm200809/cmcode/735/73502.htm

UK Parliament. (2023a). *Invisible Disabilities in Education and Employment*. https://post.parliament.uk/research-briefings/post-pn-0689

UK Parliament. (2023b). *The National Disability Strategy: Content, Reaction and Progress*. House of Commons Library. https://commonslibrary.parliament.uk/research-briefings/cbp-9599/?

Uldry, M. & EDF Women's Committee. (2022). *Forced Sterilisation of Persons with Disabilities in Europe*. European Disability Forum. www.edf-feph.org/content/uploads/2022/09/Final-Forced-Sterilisarion-Report-2022-European-Union-copia_compressed.pdf

United Nations. (1945). *United Nations Charter (full text)*. https://www.un.org/en/about-us/un-charter/full-text

United Nations. (2006). *Convention on the Rights of Persons with Disabilities*. www.un.org/disabilities/documents/convention/convention_accessible_pdf.pdf

United Nations Department of Economic and Social Affairs. (n.d.). *Factsheet on Persons with Disabilities*. www.un.org/development/desa/disabilities/resources/factsheet-on-persons-with-disabilities.html

United Nations Development Programme. (n.d.). *Disability Inclusion and Resilience*. www.undp.org/geneva/disability-inclusion-and-resilience

United Nations Office for Disaster Risk Reduction. (2023). *2023 Global Survey Report on Persons with Disabilities and Disasters*. www.undrr.org/report/2023-gobal-survey-report-on-persons-with-disabilities-and-disasters

University College London Disabled Students' Network. (2020). Disability Discrimination Faced by UCL Students & Recommended Measures. https://studentsunionucl.org/sites/default/files/u318399/documents/disabled_students_network_report.pdf

US Bureau of Labor Statistics. (2021). *Employment Situation of Disabled People*. www.bls.gov/opub/ted/2022/19-1-percent-of-people-with-a-disability-were-employed-in-2021.htm

US Bureau of Labor Statistics. (2024). *Persons with a Disability: Labor Force Characteristics Summary*. www.bls.gov/news.release/disabl.nr0.htm

US Department of Education, National Center for Education Statistics. (2020). *The Condition of Education 2020: Students with Disabilities*. https://nces.ed.gov/pubs2020/2020144.pdf

US Department of Justice. (n.d.). *Introduction to the Americans with Disabilities Act*. www.ada.gov/topics/intro-to-ada

US Department of Transportation. (2024a). *Secretary Buttigieg Announces Proposed Rule to Ensure Passengers Who Use Wheelchairs Can Fly with Dignity*. www.transportation.gov/briefing-room/secretary-buttigieg-announces-proposed-rule-ensure-passengers-who-use-wheelchairs-can

US Department of Transportation. (2024b). *Air Travel Consumer Report: June-December 2023, Full Year 2023 Airline Consumer Submissions Data*. www.transportation.gov/briefing-room/air-travel-consumer-report-june-december-2023-full-year-2023-airline-consumer

Walder, C.R. (2023, 22 September). Meet Unhidden, the fashion brand changing the game for people with disabilities. *The Guardian*. www.theguardian.com/fashion/2023/sep/21/fashion-statement-unhidden-disabled-fashion?

Wang, H. & Li, X. (2021). Privatization of healthcare in China: Trends and implications. *Chinese Health Review*, 50(1), 57–68.

Wang, K., Ostrove, J., Manning, R., Fodero, S., *et al.* (2024). Ableism in mental healthcare settings: A qualitative study among U.S. adults with disabilities. *SSM – Qualitative Research in Health*, 6, 100498. https://doi.org/10.1016/j.ssmqr.2024.100498

WebAIM. (2025). The WebAIM Million – The 2025 report on the accessibility of the top 1,000,000 home pages. https://webaim.org/projects/million

Webster, L. (2025). Primark launches clothing range designed for people with disabilities. *The Guardian*. www.theguardian.com/fashion/2025/jan/22/primark-launches-clothing-range-designed-for-people-with-disabilities

Wendell, S. (2016). *The Rejected Body: Feminist Philosophical Reflections on Disability*. Routledge.

Wheeler, E. (2022). *Three Reasons why a Disability Inclusive Workplace is a Good Idea*. AbilityNet. https://abilitynet.org.uk/news-blogs/three-reasons-why-disability-inclusive-workplace-good-idea

Williams Institute. (2021). *The Impact of the Fall 2020 COVID-19 Surge on LGBT Adults in the US*. https://williamsinstitute.law.ucla.edu/publications/covid-surge-lgbt

Williams, R. & Brownlow, S. (2016). *The Click-Away Pound Report 2016*. Freeney Williams Ltd/Click-Away Surveys Ltd. www.clickawaypound.com/downloads/cap16final2711.pdf

Wimo, A., Prince, M., & Gauthier, S. (2018). *Global Estimates of Informal Care*. Alzheimer's Disease International. www.alzint.org/resource/global-estimates-of-informal-care

Wisner, W. (2025). *11 Things About Caregiving That Nobody Warns You*. Verywell Mind. www.verywellmind.com/things-about-caregiving-8776727

Woodburn, D. & Kopić, K. (2016). *Employment of Actors with Disabilities in Television*. Ruderman Family Foundation. https://rudermanfoundation.org/white_papers/employment-of-actors-with-disabilities-in-television

World Bank. (2022). *Women, Business and the Law 2022: The Changing Landscape of Women's Economic Empowerment*. https://openknowledge.worldbank.org/entities/publication/b187725b-29ff-5c61-91e7-5110ab3c4a71

World Economic Forum. (2023). *Driving disability inclusion is more than a moral imperative – it's a business one*. www.weforum.org/stories/2023/12/driving-disability-inclusion-is-more-than-a-moral-imperative-it-s-a-business-one

World Health Organization. (n.d.a). *Disability*. www.who.int/health-topics/disability

World Health Organization. (n.d.b). Wheelchair Services. www.who.int/teams/health-product-policy-and-standards/assistive-and-medical-technology/assistive-technology/wheelchair-services

World Health Organization. (2011). *World Report on Disability*. www.who.int/publications/i/item/world-report-on-Disability

World Health Organization. (2022). *Global Report on Health Equity for Persons with Disabilities*. www.who.int/publications/i/item/9789240063600

World Health Organization & United Nations Children's Fund. (2022). *Global Report on Assistive Technology*. www.who.int/publications/i/item/9789240049451

Wright, D. (2010). *Learning Disability and the New Poor Law in England*. Taylor & Francis.

Wright, S. (2015). The historical use of aversion therapy for individuals with autism: A brief review. *Journal of the History of the Behavioral Sciences*, 51(1), 92–103.

Yale School of Public Health. (2022). Ableism cited as major barrier to mental health care for people with disabilities. *Yale Medicine News*. https://medicine.yale.edu/news-article/ableism-cited-as-major-barrier-to-mental-health-care-for-people-with-disabilities

Yin, M., Shaewitz, D., Overton, C., & Smith, D.-M. (2018). *A Hidden Market: The Purchasing Power of Working-Age Adults with Disabilities*. American Institutes for Research. www.air.org/sites/default/files/2022-03/Hidden-Market-Spending-Power-of-People-with-Disabilities-April-2018.pdf

Young, S. (2014). *I'm not your inspiration, thank you very much* [Video]. TEDxSydney. www.ted.com/talks/stella_young_i_m_not_your_inspiration_thank_you_very_much?language=en